DOES DIET CURE CANCER?

30p

DOES DIET CURE CANCER?

by

DR MAUD TRESILLIAN FERE

*Licentiate of Royal College of Physicians and Surgeons
(Edin.)
Licentiate of Royal Faculty of Physicians and Surgeons
(Glasgow)
Diploma of Public Health (London)
Tuberculosis Medical Officer: Royal Institute of Public
Health (London)*

THORSONS PUBLISHERS LIMITED
Wellingborough, Northamptonshire

First published 1963 *as*
Cancer: Its Dietetic Cause and Cure
Third Edition, revised and reset, 1971
Second Impression 1973
Third Impression 1976
Fourth Impression 1979

ISBN 0 7225 0170 6

Printed in Great Britain by
Whitstable Litho Ltd., Whitstable, Kent

CONTENTS

INTRODUCTION AND DEDICATION

The unquestioned success I have had in curing myself of cancer of the bowel has compelled me to write this book for the benefit of others.

If I seem to some readers to be 'talking down' to them, I ask them to bear with me for the sake of those who are less capable than they are of understanding. *I should also like to emphasize that the many repetitions that will be found are made with the purpose of bringing home points I wish to stress, and so cause them to be remembered.*

This book is dedicated to all cancer sufferers, and to people who strive to be well by obeying the laws of good hygiene. It is written as simply as possible so as to make its vitally important subject understood by the largest number of people.

M. T. F.

Christchurch, New Zealand.
March 1963.

ACKNOWLEDGEMENTS

The writer wishes first to express her deep gratitude and indebtedness to Doctor E. H. Smalpage, of Sydney, Australia, Fellow of the Royal College of Surgeons, England, for his research work on sodium in its relation to cancer; and also for his kind and helpful suggestions regarding two natural elements of the body, i.e. chlorine and phosphorus, being an aid in the control and elimination of excessive sodium. It is largely to his work and advice that I owe my own complete cure of cancer. His Book, *Cancer — Its Cause, Prevention and Cure,* is now, unfortunately, out of print.

CHAPTER I

HOW CANCER STARTS

We are made up of groups of an infinite number of cells of various shapes. All the cells, say, on the outside of a blood-vessel, are the same shape as each other. Those lining the inside will be of a different shape from those on the outside, but the same shape as each other. Again, those cells in the layers between will be a different shape from either, although the same as each other.

Each little cell is a tiny globe of firm jelly-like substance, and can be plainly perceived under a microscope. Some groups of cells are roundish in shape, others flat and round, others rather square or quadrangular in shape; some are even shaped like an old-fashioned soda-water bottle, with fibres coming out of the mouth. The latter sort is found in the nerve centres, as in the brain. Other cells are flattish and star-shaped, with rather an irregular number of arms; some are shaped rather like a grain of wheat, others scale-like and others are elongated.

Each little cell is a miniature person, as it were. It takes in nourishment and casts out waste matter into the fluid around it. The cell grows, increases in size, and it multiplies by a very simple and rapid method of division before birth, and a slower and more elaborate method of division after birth. This is a good thing or we would all become giants. The cell has some power of irritability; that is, the property of responding by some change to the influence of an external agent or stimulus. Apply a weak acid to the cells and their growth is checked; apply a weak alkaline solution and they are stimulated to grow faster.

It is important to emphasize that the composition of the cells before birth is much simpler than their composition after birth.

Now, normal protoplasm cells are bound together in groups by fibrous connective tissue. These with a bony frame, the skeleton, as a support, go to form the living human body.

Living material is in a state of continually unstable chemical equilibrium, building itself up on the one hand, and breaking down on the other; i.e. building simple compounds into complex compounds, and breaking down complex compounds into simple ones. The term used for the sum total of these intramolecular rearrangements is called 'metabolism'.

The health of our body cells is particularly dependent on the regular supply of one important ingredient for their nourishment, in the shape of oxygen, brought to them in the blood from the lungs; and their own regular and efficient output of the important waste matter known as carbon dioxide. Some of this acid-forming carbon dioxide waste matter is got rid of by our lungs. But most of it is neutralized by forming a compound with some alkali in our blood or tissues, and it is finally washed away through the medium of the kidneys and bladder. The alkali is generally sodium, which is present in the fluids of the body in greater quantity than any other alkali. Therefore, the *correct* amount of sodium is good for our well-being.

Here I must emphasize that an excess of sodium can be dangerous, because the excess is apt to form caustic soda, an irritant, when we are run down in health. I shall show later how sodium is a key factor in the cause of cancer.

The study of the make-up of the living body and the chemical changes which take place in the body is called Biochemistry, and it is a pity that more of it is not taught in our schools in place of much that is less important to our well-being. Now, scientists who practise biochemistry have noted the effect on the living cells of the alkalinity or acidity of the fluid surrounding each cell (the intracellular fluid).

Experiment with a Marine Cell

In an experiment it was found that if a live marine cell was placed in balanced sea-water, its division (i.e. multiplication) takes place at a certain rate. If, however, 1 in 1,000 parts of sodium chloride (i.e. table salt) is added to the sea-water the cell multiplies at an increased rate. If a mild alkaline substance is added to make the water even more alkaline, the multiplication of the cells takes place still more quickly. On the other hand, if a mild acid-producing substance, such as calcium chloride, 1 in 1,000, is added to the sea-water the rate of multiplication of the marine cell is checked or even stopped. Other mild acids added to the liquid will also check or stop the multiplication of the marine cell. Haliburton's *Handbook of Physiology* (a standard work) states that mild alkalies stimulate our cells, whereas mild acids depress the cells. Of course, very strong acids or alkalies would cauterize the cells.

The significance of such experiments is very great, indeed, in considering the cause of cancer, for similar phenomena take place in the cells of the human body. This explains why good results are obtained in the treatment of cancer by frequent, mild doses of inorganic, well-diluted acids, as hydrochloric acid, and minute doses of phosphoric acid, *which are normal in the human body;* but in cancer they are in short supply. This will be discussed at length later.

Mr. E. McDonald, of a U.S.A. Cancer Research Association, said in the American *Journal of Pharmacy,* No.607,

'The cancer cell is simply an ordinary body cell compelled to live in a wrong environment, which is due to an excess of alkalinity with a low content of calcium. Irradiation treatment, i.e. X-rays, is successful in so far as it reduces the excessive alkalinity of the blood'.

He is not the only scientist to say this, yet many medical men persist in dealing with the cells and quite ignore the quality of the fluid surrounding them. It is the abnormal quality of the fluid surrounding normal cells that irritates them to grow abnormally quickly and so form lumps.

It is well known that there is always an increased alkalinity of the plasma of the blood and body serum in cancer; and, *especially in the fluid surrounding a cancerous tumour.* This is exactly what one would expect in a body that has an abnormal amount of sodium.

How Cancer Originates

Now let us consider more closely the process of cell multiplication. The cells of the body of the infant before birth not only grow faster than after birth, but they are of a more simple structure. The fact is that when the cells in any spot in the human being start to grow abnormally fast, at the same rate as that of a pre-birth infant, they are also of the same simple internal structure.

It is this similarity in structure that the doctor looks for in the pathological laboratory when he is examining a piece of tumour under the microscope. If he finds that the cells have the same structure as those of the pre-birth infant, the verdict is 'It is malignant — it is a cancer'. The surgeon will probably say, then, that he should cut it out, if he can do so without destroying life, on the operating table. He seems to ignore the fact that a body that has one cancer tumour frequently has others which are inaccessible.

Every part of our body is supplied by nerves from the involuntary centres in the brain. When someone flicks a thing in front of one's eyes, quicker than lightning the involuntary centre in the brain causes the eyelid to shut as a sort of protective gesture. In a similar manner, when the body cells are irritated by caustic soda, produced by the action of excessive sodium, their involuntary centres in the brain seem to bid them to multiply at a greater rate so as to produce quickly lactic acid to neutralize the caustic soda. Therefore, cancer tumour formation is really an effort of the body to protect itself against the caustic soda (NaOH), because, in multiplying, the body cells always throw out lactic acid, which, as I have said, neutralizes some of the alkaline sodium.

Normally, the stomach seizes a good deal of the chlorine of table salt (salt is 50 per cent sodium and 50 per cent chlorine) to digest proteins, and the bereft sodium (which will never stay by itself for an instant) immediately seizes some of the carbon dioxide given off by the body cells, and flows round in the blood as a harmless carbonate of soda. Carbonate of soda, however, is very unstable, and, sometimes, when in excess, for reasons which will be explained later, it breaks up, and deposits the pure sodium which, when there is no acid present for it to combine with, will, we again emphasize, join some of the water moisture present to form caustic soda. This, as we have learned, so irritates the body cells that they start to multiply more quickly than normal to form lactic acid, which protects them for the time being from some of the caustic soda. Trouble arises, however, when caustic soda forms in a quantity greater than the amount of protective lactic acid present.

Lactic acid joins with sodium to form a harmless lactate salt, which is washed away by the kidneys and leaves the body via the urine.

The foregoing comprises a simple and concise explanation of how cancer has its origin in the cells of the human body.

As I have mentioned, our body cells before birth multiply very quickly by simple division. After birth, the body cells divide and multiply much more slowly by a much more elaborate manner of division. If the cells of a tumour multiply by the post-birth relatively slower manner, any lump formed is called a 'simple' tumour; and the cells of which it is composed will be seen under a microscope to be of the same composition as the cells of any human being after birth. Simple tumours do not go on increasing in size indefinitely but come to a full stop, and may never grow any bigger. But if the irritation continues and is intense enough, the cells of simple tumours may start to develop at the pre-birth rate of division, when they will show the simple form of composition of a pre-birth cell, which is called embryonic. These characteristics can be distinguished under a microscope in the pathological laboratory, and such a tumour is labelled 'malignant,' which it is.

As I have said before, the body cells of similar shape keep to their own little group. They also manifest the same characteristic in a simple tumour. Not so in a malignant tumour, where there is a proper mix-up — the cells of one shape forming tentacles into the mass of cells of another shape, creating an outline which may be likened to the limbs of an octopus. If, however, the cells of a tumour are found to have grown by the quick pre-birth manner, and are of the simple structure of the cells of a human embryo, it is called a malignant tumour, i.e. a cancer, as I have described earlier.

Objections to Biopsy

The procedure of cutting out a bit of a tumour and having it examined is called Biopsy. This procedure sounds quite good. But an increasing number of prominent scientific medical men have condemned biopsy. They say that by excising a piece of a tumour, it will be irritated, so that a simple tumour may start multiplying at pre-birth rate and so become malignant. Another objection is the fact, they say, that where a specimen of a tumour has been sent to two different laboratories, the reports have been quite opposite. They are not then quite sure what is the best to do — cut it out, or leave it *in situ*. Another criticism of biopsy is that it often causes metastasis of the primary malignant tumour to other parts of the body. Metastasis is a medical term to express a theory that there is always *one* malignant tumour to start with, and that any other malignant tumour, in that patient, spreads from the first tumour through the lymphatics or the blood-vessels. The theory is based on the fact that where there are several malignant tumours in one patient, they consist of all *one shape of cells*, no matter how many tumours there are, or where they are placed. We rely on the pathological laboratories for this statement. Late in the disease, it is said, there may sometimes be different-shaped cells affected.

All medical scientists do not accept the theory of metastasis. One medical scientist calls it an 'economy of effort of Nature'. I think he is right. For instance, when one flicks his eyelid involuntarily to protect his eyes, he does not, at the same time, draw up, say, his leg. The surgeons who believe in metastasis seem to ignore the quality of the fluids of the body; and also the influence of these fluids on the body cells. They also seem to ignore the influence of the control of the subconscious part of the brain, and the influence of the reaction of the numerous nerve fibres around the various cells of our body. The nerve fibres from one shape of body cell will all stem from the particular nerve centre in the brain; or from one set of nerve centres in the brain that are all closely connected. Therefore, any recurrence of the tumour would be formed of the same-shaped body cells, although not formed of a piece of the original tumour.

CHAPTER II

A KNOWLEDGE OF BIOCHEMISTRY

In order that readers may understand more clearly the subject of biochemistry as it affects the purpose of this book, I ask them to study the following simple explanation. Whenever I may repeat anything I have said before, it is done simply for the sake of emphasis and easy memorizing.

Pure water is formed of a molecule consisting of two atoms of hydrogen and one of oxygen. An element is a substance that consists of all one sort of thing. All the minerals are elements.

The smallest particle of an element is called an atom, and the compound of two or more atoms in a liquid is called a molecule.

We have a large number of alkaline and acid elements in the make-up of our body's economy. Important among them are sodium, potassium, calcium, magnesium, manganese, iron, copper, iodine, phosphorus, chlorine, and sulphur. The last four are of an acid-producing nature, and so they help to prevent excessive alkalinity, which too much of the others would tend to produce.

Alkaline and Acid Balance

The great need for health is perfect balance between these two opposing elements. Most people know that acidity in our body reaction is bad, but few people realize that excess of alkalinity is equally dangerous. This overlooked scientific fact is behind the cause of cancer (*in a debilitated constitution*) as well as of at least twenty other diseases.

The inorganic acid and alkaline elements have a great attraction for each other and will always unite when they get the opportunity, as when they meet in a liquid. An equal portion of sodium and chlorine makes the compound known commonly as table salt (NaC). Because it is so tasty, far too many people take a real excess in their various articles of food and as a condiment, to their great potential detriment. There are many different salts, but as none of them is nice tasting, we are not likely to take them in excess, as we do table salt.

We can be burnt with fire or strong acids. The damage they do can be checked with a sufficient quantity of water. This is very different in the case of certain alkaline substances. As I have said, alkaline substances tend to unite with acid substances whenever they get the chance, but when there are no acid substances present for an alkaline substance, such as sodium, to unite with, and there is any water present, sodium will promptly join with the water to form a powerful caustic, namely, caustic soda (NaOH). For another illustration, calcium in its compound of unslaked lime will form a burning fluid substance when water is added. Men working with it often receive bad burns, say, on the hands. But immediately they add some acid, even vinegar, it eases them, because alkalies love acids more than water.

This chemical fact is the basis of the dietetic treatment for cancer, as outlined later. Weakened hydrochloric acid is used to neutralize the caustic soda formation in the body. The body, when it is in a debilitated condition, is incapable of neutralizing an excess of sodium.

If a chemist extracts some pure sodium from its

compound, sodium chloride (table salt), he has to keep the sodium by itself, in, say, a glass jar, under naphtha, with which it does not happen to have any affinity.

A chemistry master may one day take his class into the chemical laboratory and select two boys to demonstrate that, if sodium can obtain no acids to join with, and there is water present, it will always join with the water to form caustic soda. He gives each one of the boys a little lump of pure sodium and bids them drop it into a little basin of water in front of him. The sodium will rush round in the water as if it were alive, and, if a large enough piece, it may even throw out sparks. (Not a nice thing to have in your body, you will think.) A faint vapour rises off the top of the water. What is happening? The pure sodium is tearing the molecules of water to pieces and it is forming caustic soda. Thus, you see, sodium is, indeed, a very active substance and it is very powerful.

A substance extracted from certain vegetables, called litmus, will dye paper red. If a piece of this red litmus paper is dipped into an alkaline liquid it will turn various shades of blue, according to the concentration of alkali in the solution. If you dip a piece of this red paper into a basin of plain water, it will not change colour; but if you dip it in after a lump of sodium has been dropped in the water, the red paper will turn blue, which shows the water has become alkaline. (Litmus paper can be procured from any chemist's shop for a few pence.)

As I have explained before, we are made up of myriads of little particles, called cells. We take food to provide nourishment for these cells. Our food is turned by the process of metabolism into heat, energy, body substance, and waste matter, which waste matter is eliminated by the lungs, skin, kidneys, and bowels. Sodium, especially in its compound of sodium chloride (table salt) is a useful and necessary substance. It is only an excess which can be injurious. Many medicines are like that — good in the correct dose and dangerous in excess.

The elements which nourish our body enter into the composition of the cells of the body, whereas sodium is said to exist, normally, mostly in the *liquids* of the body. It helps to control the correct density of the fluids of the body and so enables nutriment to reach the cells, and the waste matter to be taken away. Most important is sodium's work in neutralizing acidity in the body.

Dangers of Table Salt

A chemist uses the term 'grain' for a special measure of weight. His fifteen grains equal about a quarter of a teaspoon. He calls his teaspoon (which is a definite size) a drachm. He says thirty grains would be half a drachm and sixty grains a whole drachm. One biochemist, a Dr. Estes, says we could keep quite healthy on fifteen grains of table salt per twenty-four hours; that would be about quarter of a teaspoon. Other biochemists vary a little in regard to what is the wholesome quantity. The majority of English biochemists say that we could take sixty grains of table salt per twenty-four hours, i.e. roughly one teaspoonful. It is said rather scathingly by some that the average Western individual consumes 200 to 500 grains of table salt per twenty-four hours. This would be from three to eight teaspoonfuls. Often, when I have asked a patient if she took much table salt, she would say, 'Very little, doctor. I never take more than about a quarter of a teaspoonful of table salt at table.' But she was quite surprised when I pointed out the large quantity she might be getting in the various foods she ate; in her butter, bread, and cooked foods, etc., etc., etc. Even the ancients were aware of the danger of taking an excess of table salt. We know this, because of seeing the warnings to their people on some of their old tablets.

As regards meat, one biochemist has a little joke. He says, 'Raw meats contain a good deal of sodium, but it is neutralized and rendered harmless by the chlorine and phosphorus meat also contains. But when it is cooked, the chlorine and phosphorus evaporate and leave the sodium'. 'So,' he says, 'you would be quite safe if you ate it raw!'

Bakers put a lot of table salt into their bread to make it tasty. One baker put nine pounds of table salt every day into the bread he made from four sacks of white flour, which turned out a few hundred loaves. Factory-produced butter is said to contain as much as about half a teaspoon of table salt to every ounce of butter. Most tinned meat and similar products contain table salt, not only to make them tasty, but also because table salt is a helpful preservative. There is sodium in many chemist's tablets, especially aspirin tablets. Think of the quantity of aspirin tablets consumed! Even ice cream often contains table salt. Think of the thousands of recipes which finish up with the direction, 'Add so much table salt', usually from a quarter to one teaspoonful. Beer and stout are said to contain some table salt. Cheese, bacon, salt beef, sausages, saveloys, and such-like meat products, contain table salt. Fish has its own content of salt. There is also plenty in gravy powders and flavourings. Nearly every cook uses quantities of table salt for cooking vegetables. Further, due to overcooking or using an excess of water or too high a cooking temperature vegetables lose their natural flavour, and so salt for flavour is added, as a matter of course.

It is important to remember, too, that sodium in combination with sulphur is frequently used by butchers and fishmongers in far too large a quantity for our health, for its antiseptic and preservative qualities; but not so much since they have had refrigeration.

Some people, when they experience acidity in the stomach, put half a teaspoon of sodium bicarbonate ($NaHCO_3$) in half a cup of water and drink it, and they say they experience relief. A faintly acid gas rises at once in their mouth. What has happened? 2 $NaHCO_3$ (sodium bicarbonate) equals 2 $NaOH$ (caustic soda) plus 2 CO_2 (carbonic dioxide gas) which gas rises up in their mouth. The $NaOH$ (caustic soda), which is a strong alkali, promptly unites with the acidity in the stomach, which is the cause of their trouble, and they get relief.

There are two main branches of chemistry:

1. Inorganic Chemistry. (Inorganic means not organic.) This deals with simple substances and their compounds. The simple substances are elements. An element is a substance that consists of only one sort of thing. All the minerals are elements. But all the elements are not minerals, as : (N) Nitrogen; (H) Hydrogen; (O) Oxygen; (C) Carbon.

2. The second branch of chemistry is known as Organic Chemistry. The word 'organic' signifies organized. It deals with compound substances. These substances have been manufactured in the make-up of some living thing, such as plant or animal.

Carbon dioxide given off by our body cells is an organic substance. If joined with a molecule of water it forms carbonic acid — thus : $CO_2 + H_2O = H_2CO_3$ i.e. carbonic acid.

3. Apart from the two branches just described, there is a third group called Synthetic Compounds. These are often very complicated and are made up by the chemists in imitation, very often, of organic compounds which they claim to better. There are, unfortunately, a great number of these synthetic compounds. Advertisements of them are

sent constantly to hospitals, chemists, and doctors, in which they are alleged to provide a cure for one complaint or another. This may be true; but, unfortunately, they do not say anything, as a rule, about their reaction or side-effects, or their after-effects, which are often very injurious. The synthetic compounds are done up in an innumerable array of tablets, capsules, etc., or fluids ready for hypodermic injection. The poor patient in hospital has no chance at all; if he tries to avoid swallowing the tablets he will just get a shot from a hypodermic syringe.

Drugs Can Kill

In my opinion there are far too many of these tablets given in our public hospitals. I had a young man patient who was getting on very nicely on my constitutional treatment, when I was rung up one morning to be told that he had had some slight accident and had been sent into the public hospital. I went down next morning to see him. I said to the Sister of the ward, 'What particular drugs are you giving him?' She told me. I said, 'That's all right — I am glad you are not giving him any C—, which is an antibiotic.' I added, 'You know, Sister, a good many patients have died because of that wretched drug.' Sister said, 'Well, the doctors must have somebody to experiment on.' 'And who would be a guinea pig?' I asked facetiously. She did not reply.

A big cause of the present failure to remove or prevent cancer is that both the people and far too many doctors concentrate on symptoms instead of the causes of most diseases. People may go to their doctor complaining of pain or aches or tiredness or nervousness or headaches, or indigestion, or constipation, or sleeplessness, or palpitation, and the doctor may apply to their trouble a mysterious name and give them some tablets. They might be quite offended if the doctor asked them about their bad habits, or the breaking of any of the Ten Commandments of Good Health, which are enumerated in Chapter XVIII.

CHAPTER III

THE ACIDITY-ALKALINITY BALANCE

Good health is maintained by our having a correct balance between the reaction of the two opposite inorganic elements — the acid and alkaline ones. And the main thing is 'Correct Quantity is as important as Quality.' If you will turn to my diagram (on page 18) of a pendulum in an inverted V, you will see that I have tried to show the relative elements as they affect the correct reaction of our blood and body in good health. On the right-hand side the alkaline elements are noted.

Let us consider the alkaline elements. Sodium in its normal quantity exists largely in the liquid of the body; but when it is in great excess it tends to enter the body cells themselves and turn calcium out. This has a weakening effect on the muscular strength and action. We note, in consequence, that the cancer patient generally has weakly acting bowels because the muscles of the intestines are depleted of their calcium content. Hence, most cancer patients suffer greatly from constipation. In heart conditions, excessive sodium may add to the trouble by depleting the cells of the cardiac muscles of their calcium, and thereby causing a weakening of the heart's beat.

I have noted, for more than twenty years, i.e. since I have been especially concerned with cancer, that is, after my own self-cure, that the majority of cancer patients tend to have a weak pulse.

MAIN SUBSTANCES AFFECTING THE CHEMICAL BALANCE
OF THE BODY

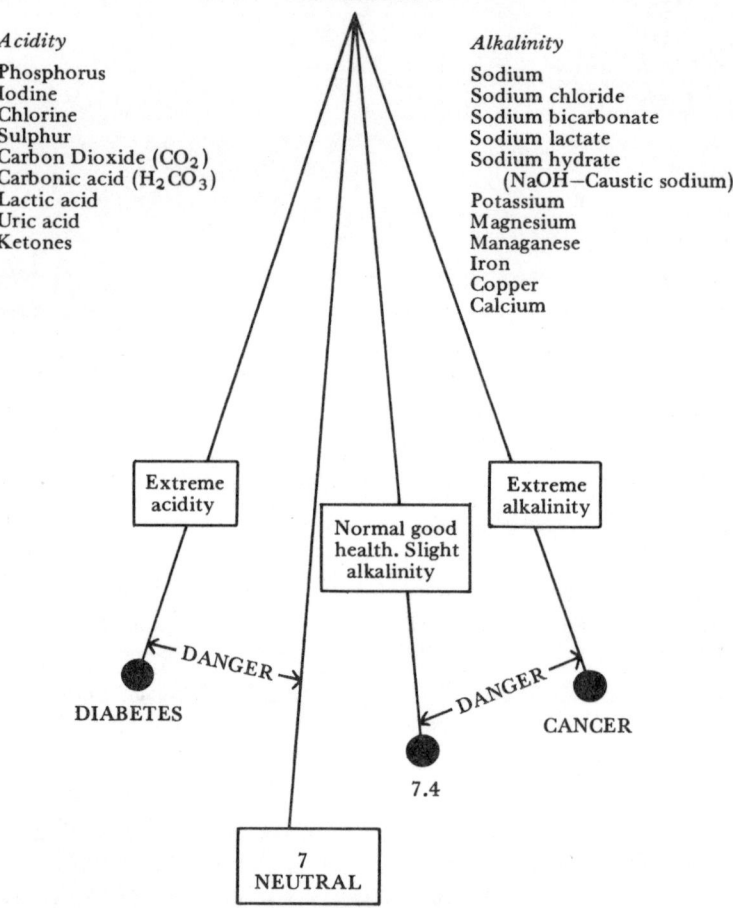

Acidity

Phosphorus
Iodine
Chlorine
Sulphur
Carbon Dioxide (CO_2)
Carbonic acid (H_2CO_3)
Lactic acid
Uric acid
Ketones

Alkalinity

Sodium
Sodium chloride
Sodium bicarbonate
Sodium lactate
Sodium hydrate
(NaOH—Caustic sodium)
Potassium
Magnesium
Managanese
Iron
Copper
Calcium

Extreme acidity

Normal good health. Slight alkalinity

Extreme alkalinity

← DANGER →

← DANGER →

DIABETES

CANCER

7.4

7
NEUTRAL

In good health our blood and lymph are slightly alkaline, as also are our bodies. Our tissues vary between acidity and alkalinity.

Our urine is mildly acid, except after a big meat meal, when it may be alkaline, because the stomach has taken so much of the chlorine out of the blood to help it digest the proteins. Animal proteins require more chlorine for their digestion than vegetable proteins, and this frees more sodium in the system. This is why it is necessary to put the sodium-affected patient on a vegetarian diet while trying to free his system of excess sodium. (Note comments on the treatment of cancer in Chapter XIX.)

Magnesium, manganese, iron, and copper are all in-organic alkaline elements concerned with the balance of the make-up of the body.

There are traces of many other elements that I have not included in the diagram. Scientists are not sure in some cases whether they are present by accident, or whether they are a necessary part of the body's make-up. Some say they are most important, and research is continuously being conducted in this field.

On the left-hand side of the diagram of the pendulum in the inverted V, the acid-making elements are noted. There is chlorine, which we need in abundance; and, in much smaller quantities, phosphorus, which is needed in the composition of the body cells. Iodine, needed in small quantities, is nevertheless very important, especially for the proper functioning of the thyroid gland. Then there is sulphur, which, among other things, helps the proper functioning of the bowels. Then there is the important little organic compound of CO_2 (carbon dioxide) pro-duced by the body cells in the expression of heat and energy.

Next is the important lactic acid, which is a stronger acid than carbon dioxide, and, as we have described earlier, is always produced by the cells when they multiply, as they do, by division.

The normal reaction of the blood is always slightly alkaline. The slightest change in its reaction is so important that scientists do not calculate it in whole figures. They take the figure seven as the reaction of pure water, which is neither acid nor alkaline. 7.4 is considered by English laboratories to be the alkaline reaction of normal blood. Some laboratories on the continent of Europe say 7.3 is the normal alkaline reaction, and, again, some American laboratories say 7.5. Anything below 7.3 is called acidosis, although the *blood* may not be acid at all. The reaction seldom registers the neutral seven.

I have indicated by the pendulum the dangerous position of excessive alkalinity.

Normal urine is always slightly acid, except for a short while after, say, a big meal, when the stomach has taken an extra amount of chlorine from the blood to help digest the meat. Our *tissues* vary between slightly acid and slightly alkaline. The liver is a great controlling organ, and is very important in its beneficial action with regard to our health. People should consider the welfare of their liver a great deal more than they do. It is especially important in treating a cancer patient to study the liver all the time, and see that one does not overburden it in any way.

The problem of the system's acidity/alkalinity balance rests almost wholly on the basis of the food we eat.

Few people realize that wrong food contributes towards the production of cancer as well as many other diseases, and that cancer cannot be checked unless the right food is eaten in the correct proportions. Eating unbalanced food causes irritant poisons to be formed. When you become run down in health, and consequently cannot continue to throw off irritant poisons you may become a victim to cancer, especially if you are taking an excessive amount of sodium chloride (table salt) in the food you eat, as most people do unwittingly.

Often people are not aware of the unbalance in their bodies for a considerable time, usually not until they feel that something is wrong, or they have an unusual lump somewhere. They realize, then, that they should obtain medical advice.

Cancer is a Constitutional Disease
It is no good having a bit of one's body cut out, as in a

cancer operation, if the irritant poison is in one's whole body. One must eat the right food in the right proportions and so purify the bloodstream, thus rendering any operation unnecessary.

In the ordinary operation for cancer the patient is warned to return to the surgeon for a check-up in three months' time to see if there is a recurrence of the cancer tumour, which, of course, can be expected if the irritant poison is still in his system. No doubt it will be if he has not cleansed his system by a purifying diet and strict obedience to the Ten Commandments of Health, as well as drastically lessened the previous excessive intake of sodium.

I repeat that cancer is a constitutional disease, like rheumatism or the common cold. Therefore, it can never be permanently cured by merely cutting chips or chunks out of the body or being burnt through radium or X-rays. Irradiation by the latter two things causes the sodium carbonates to break up and create more caustic soda, which burns the body, unless washed away by the kidneys. Any sensible person knows that if one has the care of any bird, fowl, dog, cat, horse, or other animal, and one feeds them wrongly, they will soon become sick; and, if one does not correct the mistake they will die. *Why should one think that the human animal is made any differently?*

A kitten was fed on cooked meat with a high salt content. In three months it developed a cancer tumour. Then it was fed on raw meat and in a few months the cancer disappeared. We know that sailors, who eat a lot of salt meat, are very prone to cancer. Many people have rotted their natural teeth by the habitual use of deficient, wrong foods, or wrong habits of eating, and then they obtain artificial teeth to continue the sad process of health degeneration. It is sad to realize that the great majority of people eat merely what they think tastes nice, or even just what looks nice, regardless of its health value.

On visiting a fowl farm recently, I noticed some of the birds had lost many tail feathers. One or two had an ulcerated patch on the bare part under a wing. The proprietor told me he noticed frequent lumps on the birds' insides when he was cleaning them for sale, and that he was quite aware that these lumps were caused by the table salt that he put into their bran mash. He said, however, that he was a business man and not a philanthropist. And he said also that the table salt made the fowls lay well. I suggested that quantity could be a factor, and if he put in a little less table salt, the birds would be even more fit, and perhaps lay even more. I fear that my solicitation on behalf of the birds fell on deaf ears, but it is interesting to note how excessive salt can affect birds as well as human beings.

A clever London doctor once persuaded a sick and overfed patient, suffering badly from indigestion, to put into a basin similar amounts of everything he ate for one day; and at the end of the day to have a good look into the basin. The patient then realized what awful mixtures his stomach had had to tackle, and no longer wondered why he had digestive troubles.

When a grown-up person goes to a medical man with similar symptoms from the same causes, i.e. eating excessively of rich food — the medical man may say, 'Here is something to stop the pain and I will give you something else to stop the diarrhoea and vomiting.' 'Wonderful doctor,' says the patient, 'one dose and he stopped my pain.' The patient's fermenting belly mess is therefore nicely retained, and so he is in that medical man's care for months.

Oh! this is the Age of Symptom Suppressing! Of course,

such symptomatic treatment is really not very ethical, nor at all scientific; but why blame the medical man? Demand creates the supply. The medical man has got to earn his living under the present stupid system. No treatment can ever be really permanently efficient, unless the patient himself will do things — firstly, deny himself certain things, which many patients very much dislike doing; and exercise self-control and self-direction. Secondly — to think for himself about his body and his health, again disliked by many patients.

CHAPTER IV

OUR PERSONAL CHEMICAL LABORATORY

It is fortunate that sodium prefers to unite with acids rather than water; although, when there are no acids present, it will unite with water and form caustic soda, the surplus hydrogen rising as a light vapour off the water. It is the hydrogen atom for which the sodium atom had no use. Thus, our body's chemical laboratory goes to great trouble to prevent or neutralize and eliminate any dangerous compounds of excessive sodium.

Someone has said that our bodies are slow-combustion engines; but it would be equally correct to say that we are chemical laboratories which are continually building up simple compounds into complicated ones, and breaking down complicated substances into simple compounds, in the processes of producing heat, energy and body substance. In normal, healthy persons, it is true that some sodium compounds neutralize some excessive acidity in the body, and in that way, and if not in *excessive* amount, they are of good use to our health.

Acid-Forming Foods to Avoid

To attain good health, if suffering from acidity, it is best to avoid any excess of acid-forming foods, such as devitalized white bread, with its bleaching powders, and also too much sugar of all kinds, especially cane sugar and any excess of treacle or golden syrup. Take honey not more often than twice a week. Avoid meat, game, poultry,

fish, particularly shell fish, and too much fat; fried fatty
things, especially when permeated with fat, are very bad.
They all have a worse action in the hot weather. Eggs
should only be eaten every second day, as it takes the liver
forty-eight hours to finish dealing with an egg. After fifty
years of age, and, indeed, after forty years with many
people, it would be best to have flesh meat not more often
than once a week. Vegetable proteins, which consist of
nuts and legumes, should be taken daily. A fact everyone
should know is that all starch has to be turned into body
sugar by our liver before it can be of use to our body; and
all sugar and sweet stuff also has to be turned into body
sugar before it can be of use to our body. Therefore, you
can see what an important organ our liver is, and how
careful we should be not to overwork 'it.

Our kidneys are always trying to purify the blood
circulating through them, by excreting any acid, so that is
why the urine from any normal body is slightly acid. Dip a
piece of red litmus paper into such urine, and it does not
change colour. Before taking any chlorine-acid treatment
for cancer, the urine of a *cancer patient* will generally turn
red litmus paper blue. The red litmus paper only turns blue
in the presence of an *alkaline* substance. We know the
compound of ammonia is alkaline, and that it is very
volatile, that is, it easily evaporates into a gas. Wave a piece
of red litmus paper over the mouth of a bottle of
ammonia, and watch it turn blue. Ammonia is a much
milder alkali than is sodium hydrate (caustic soda).

To return to our examination of sodium, the question
of whether it is good or bad in our body depends on the
quantity. In the correct amount it is good. In *excess* it is
dangerous. The vital point is to know what is the correct
amount. There is, unfortunately, a considerable *variation*
in what different individuals can take, with seeming

impunity. Further, in different states of temperature and physical exertion, the desirable quantities of sodium that can be taken will vary considerably. The hotter the temperature and the greater the exertion the bigger the amount of sodium that can be taken, with, of course, the appropriate increase of water intake. Also, in certain diseases, such as in a certain stage of Addison's disease, a big intake of sodium in its compound of table salt, often seems to be of great benefit.

Menace of Excessive Sodium

We must realize, too, that habit can be an important factor. We know that a person who has accustomed himself to some dangerous poison, such as opium or arsenic, can often take, with seeming impunity, as much of the poison in one day as would kill ten ordinary persons, who had not so accustomed themselves to the imbibing of the poison. But that is not to say that people who take poison with apparent impunity will always be able to do so. It is a fact well known to scientists that, all of a sudden, without any recognized warning, the poison the person is taking, quite harmlessly to date, will suddenly take poisonous action, and make him very ill, or even kill him. It seems as if the body has been working under a strain and suddenly goes on strike. But it does not seem to me that it could have been so sudden as appeared at first sight. No doubt there were lots of warning symptoms, if there had been anyone wise enough to recognize them.

Tobacco smoking, and using sodium in any of its compounds, in excess, fall into the same category as those poisons. Remember how easy it is to take sodium to excess via table salt in a multiplicity of foods; especially salt butter with its dangerous amount of half a teaspoon of table salt to the ounce. Remember that British biochemists are agreed that the normal person does not require more than a teaspoon of table salt as a *maximum* per twenty-four hours distributed in all one's food, as in butter, cheese, bread, cooked food, etc. And some think an even less amount should be the minimum. It is a never-failing source of wonder to me that *the menace of excessive sodium* has been so overlooked. If I said to you, 'I have a theory that if I put my hands in water they will get wet,' you would be quite justified in retorting, 'Do not be ridiculous, that is no theory.' Well, that is my attitude to cancer and excessive sodium as its cause in a body that has ceased to tolerate the excess.

CHAPTER V

PHOSPHORUS AND CHLORINE

The ordinary cancer patient who comes to me, and who fulfils my one great requirement — *co-operation* — for three months, experiences great relief from pain, and is generally enabled to dispense in three weeks with the pain-killing drugs he has been taking. This, of course, makes a great impression on the patient and his friends. Further, my practice of placing a piece of red litmus paper on the outside of the upper gum of a patient for from two to three minutes to obtain a *rough* estimate of whether they tend to suffer from alkalinity or acidity of their tissues, as estimated by the blue discolouring of the paper in alkalinity, has been most helpful. When one member of a family has cancer, and the whole family try the litmus paper test, the difference between the blue colour reaction of the patient and the reaction of the other members of the family is most marked, and so, of course, they are greatly impressed.

As the family has been eating more or less the same food — and more or less been making the same mistakes — one would, perhaps, not expect such a marked difference. We must realize here that the body of the cancer patient, for various reasons connected with disobedience of the Commandments of Good Health, has ceased to have the ability to cope with the excess of sodium, for no longer has he the vitality to neutralize and eliminate it.

Let us now consider phosphorus. It is a very powerful

acid-forming element, and although it exists only in a tiny amount in our normal body, that amount is very important to our health. Phosphorus enters into the composition of our body cells.

If the patient took the British Pharmacopoeia regulated strength of the weak, liquid, phosphoric acid, called Acid Phosphoricum Dilutum, he would have a medicine in which there are ten drops of Acid Phosphoricum Dilutum in a teaspoon of liquid, which would correspond to the one-fiftieth of a grain dose that is prescribed in a pill by Dr. Smalpage. I prescribe the liquid dose, with two tablespoons of water (as I cannot obtain the pills), after meals, three times a day, during the first two months of treatment. Many patients declare they experience relief with it. For identification I colour this phosphorus mixture pink with a couple of drops of liquid extract of amaranth, which is a harmless vegetable extract. *It should be noted carefully that if the patient is having chlorine in the form of Pulvis Calcium Chloride, in capsules, he cannot have any phosphorus at the same time, for chemical reasons.* You would have to depend in such a case on the patient obtaining sufficient phosphorus in his raw fruit and vegetable salad; or, alternatively, the phosphorus and calcium should be given at least a couple of hours apart.

Organized Phosphorus

Phosphorus is normally used by our body to help neutralize excess of sodium. It is in short supply in cases of cancer, which is because the patient has neglected to take sufficient phosphorus-containing foods, in the form of raw fruit and vegetable salads. These foods, containing organized phosphorus, are the safest method of giving this useful but very dangerous substance when given in excess of the body's requirement. Therefore, I have always discouraged cancer patients from continuing with the phosphorus medicine after the first two months' treatment; though they sometimes persuade me to continue giving it for a few weeks longer, as they declare it helps them. If it is really desirable to continue giving phosphorus, I prefer to give it in the third month and afterwards through the medium of one teaspoon of Parrish's chemical food, in a little water, once or twice a day, after meals. This is useful because it also contains iron and calcium, two necessary substances always deficient in the cancer patient. There is one thing Parrish's chemical food is short of, however, and that is copper sulphate, which is so helpful to the absorption of iron; therefore, I get a grain of copper sulphate added to an eight-ounce bottle of Parrish's chemical food.

Now, if the patient cannot chew raw salads, he can always take them finely chopped or minced, or put through a pulverizing machine, or mixer.

Here note for future reference that the skins of some vegetables contain a good deal of what may be termed a 'hot' condiment, similar to red pepper, and this can be very irritating if taken in excess, in raw juices. The skin of white turnips is one such instance. We must study and know the subject of correct diet; without which we cannot have good health. When table salt is reduced in order to free the patient of his excessive sodium, he must not go short of the important mineral, iodine, which in some countries is added to some brands of table salt. Many people, knowing this, deliberately take a dangerous excess of table salt so as to obtain the precious iodine. You will see, in the treatment chapter, how I made sure of having the minim a day of the precious iodine.

There is another most important biochemical element, chlorine, of which the cancer patient tends to be short. Table salt, as you now know well, is 50 per cent chlorine and 50 per cent sodium, and so in cutting down on table salt to lessen excessive sodium, the patient should not be deprived of the vital chlorine. Therefore, I made sure of obtaining it freely, as will be seen in Chapter XIX.

Chlorine is necessary to the stomach to digest protein food. It is also a very important neutralizer of sodium. This I have experienced personally. I consider it was the chief thing which saved my life, *as far as medicines go,* when I myself was afflicted with cancer. Of course, I have a good knowledge of diet, and a good working knowledge of the laws of true hygiene. The application of these was a vital factor in the successful treatment of cancer in my own case. Indeed, they are vital factors in the successful treatment of all diseases. It is regrettable that they are too often ignored by medical men and their patients.

CHAPTER VI

A BRIEF SURVEY OF CHEMICAL FACTORS

In the cancer patient there is an excess of carbonate of soda, causing an increase of the very slight natural alkalinity of the blood. There is a deficiency of blood phosphates and chlorides, which are acid-forming and so neutralize the alkaline sodium compounds. In the urine there is a complete absence of the usual urinary acid-forming phosphates and chlorides. Any layman can prove the loss of the normal acidity of the urine by dropping a leaf of red litmus paper into urine passed first thing in the morning, and watch it turn blue, as red litmus paper always does in the presence of an alkali. If the urine was from a normal healthy person, the litmus paper dropped into the urine would stay red, showing that the urine was acid, as it mostly should be in good health. Of course, the urine should be only faintly acid, but if the patient should very recently have had a big meat meal, his urine may be neutral, or even slightly alkaline, because the stomach has needed extra hydrochloric acid and has taken it.

It should be noticed that the kidneys are always draining off any acid from the blood, hence the healthy normal person has a faintly acid urine, which contains some phosphates and chlorates.

Testing the Blood
Let us now consider the blood. A layman can hardly experiment with that, of course. The reaction of the blood

shows, however, to a very considerable extent in the tissues of superficial mucous membranes, where fluid oozes out of the tiny blood vessels. One such place is very accessible for testing the reaction; i.e. the outside moist surface of the upper gum. Gently press a strip of red litmus paper lengthways on the gum, and then lower the top lip. Leave for three to four minutes, and then remove the litmus paper and lay it on a piece of white paper. Note that in an *untreated* cancer patient it will, generally, have turned *very* blue; but, if the person is normal and healthy, that is, a person with no excess of the alkali sodium in his system, the red litmus paper will be a faint mauve, or only a very slight pale blue in parts, chiefly only on the edges. In order to show that litmus paper turns blue in the presence of an alkali, take a typical alkaline liquid, such as a half-teaspoon of sodium bicarbonate in half a cup of water, and dip the red litmus paper in it. You will find that it turns blue in the solution.

Never forget that there are two sets of elements in the body, the acid elements and the alkaline elements, and that they neutralize each other. There are many compound (organic) substances in the body that are acid or alkaline. Those we have to consider are lactic acid and uric acid. Sometimes there are also bad organic acids, such as half-digested fats, called Ketones, and these are sometimes found even in an alkaline blood. As I have indicated, these compound substances belong to the organic group of chemistry. Partaking of an excess of animal fat is said to produce ketones. Organic compounds are said to generally have one or more atoms of carbon in their make-up.

Oxygen Essential for Red Corpuscles
Once an organic substance is broken up, we cannot generally put the same particles together again in the same

way. Also note that in cancer, there is a great deficiency of oxyhaemoglobin. This is the substance in the red corpuscles of the blood that carries the carbon dioxide (thrown off by the body cells) to the lungs, where it is exchanged for oxygen, which they (the red corpuscles) bring back again from the lungs to the body cells, which are each a slow combustion engine. A normal body cell burns and gives off heat and energy, and like any other combustion engine, it gives off carbon dioxide (CO_2). The oxyhaemoglobin in the little red blood corpuscles is the substance that enables them to seize some of this CO_2, and when the corpuscles return again in the blood to the lungs, they swap the CO_2 for oxygen, which they then carry back in the circulation to the body cells; again swapping for a particle of CO_2, which the body cells are continuously giving off.

The foregoing cycle or performance, call it what you will, is the very essence of our life. If there was no oxygen in our lungs for the red corpuscles to obtain we would not live long, if the absence of oxygen lasted for more than a very few minutes.

There are many degrees between the total withholding of oxygen and the blood corpuscles continuously being supplied with their perfect quota of oxygen. Several factors may come into action. The very important and most obvious one is that if the corpuscle went to the lungs without its particle of CO_2 it would receive no oxygen.

Then there is another cycle going on all the time, the one I have been explaining repeatedly, and that is the action of the sodium atom in seizing a CO_2 particle, and forming with it a non-irritating compound, a carbonate of sodium, which flows round in the blood quite harmlessly.

The biochemists speak of this latter group of CO_2 as the *combined* carbon dioxide; and the CO_2 which the red corpuscles carry to the lungs as the *free* carbon dioxide. A very important quotation is taken from a standard work on biochemistry, *Acidosis and Alkalosis,* by Graham and Morris (E. & S. Livingstone, Edinburgh). These two doctor-scientists, one-time lecturers on biochemistry at the University of Glasgow, Scotland, say :

'Anything which increases the ratio of free carbon dioxide to combined carbon dioxide will result in an acidosis; and, conversely, anything which diminishes the ratio of free carbon dioxide to combined carbon dioxide will result in an alkalosis.'

Please study carefully that statement, because it puts in a nutshell what I might write pages about, and not express so clearly and convincingly. Most people are well aware of the danger of acidosis; but many people, both doctors and patients, ignore, or are unaware of, the menace of excessive alkalinity. The chief point I wish to make is that for perfect health there must be the perfect balance, that is, the perfect ratio between two cycles : (1) the cycle of the red corpuscle with carbon dioxide, with its swift movement, and (2) the cycle of the sodium with its combining with carbon dioxide to flow round in the blood-stream as a carbonate of sodium.

You will note that I speak of a carbonate of sodium as if there were several varieties, well so there are. But for the purpose of this book that is immaterial.

Cancer Patients Lack Oxygen

In cancer there is too much of the alkali sodium for the good action of the little red corpuscles in bringing oxygen from the lungs to the body cells. Some of them are deprived of their quota of CO_2 by the excess of sodium, so they have nothing to swap for oxygen when in the blood-stream they reach the lungs. Therefore, the cancer patient does not obtain enough oxygen. Nothing can burn properly without oxygen — neither fires, lamps, candles, matches, nor our body cells. Anybody who does not get enough fresh air (oxygen) tends to become very anaemic. The pallor and deadly anaemia of advancing cancer patients is a matter of common observation. We know tubercular patients often have bouts of temperature : they burn too fast. Not so the cancer patient — he feels the cold because he tends to burn too slowly; he lacks oxygen. His whole system tends to get run down, his pulse tends to be slower and less vigorous than normal. He generally suffers from sluggish action of the bowels. Because his circulation is poor, he tends to have chronically cold feet and hands. He tends to be listless and easily tired. Now, the degree and severity of these symptoms depends entirely on the amount of excess sodium and the degree of vitality the body has to cope with it.

There are cases where the vitality is very low and there is a great excess of sodium. In consequence, too many of the red corpuscles are permanently deprived of their quota of CO_2 and, therefore, of their portion of oxygen. This has such a bad effect on the little red corpuscles that many of them suddenly perish. They die and so become foreign matter in the blood-stream. Then the leucocytes try to remove them by exercising their function of phagocytosis, and we have the condition known as Leukaemia. This is, as I have said, a fatal form of cancer, where the patient may die in a few days. It is especially malignant in little children, where the mother's blood has had an excess of sodium, and so the baby is born with an excess of sodium. Then, if the baby is artificially fed, and his milk bottles have been cleaned by the dairyman with a caustic soda solution, and not properly rinsed, the result is disastrous. The amount of caustic soda thus transmitted may be very small in amount, it is true, but dangerous for the baby, who has already too much sodium in his system from his mother's blood before he was born.

CHAPTER VII

SIGNS OF CANCER

The members of the New Zealand Branch of the British Empire Cancer Campaign give the following as the Seven Danger Signs of Cancer:

1. Any sore that does not heal.
2. A lump or thickening in the breast or elsewhere.
3. Unusual bleeding or discharge.
4. Any change in a wart or mole.
5. Persistent indigestion or difficulty in swallowing.
6. Persistent hoarseness or cough.
7. Any change in normal bowel habits.

The following are other signs of possible cancer that I have noted in my long career as a doctor :

1. Pain on breathing, especially deeply, with no increased temperature, might suggest cancer of the lungs, especially in the case of a heavy smoker.
2. When the patient complains of a burning pain in some place and you put your hand on the part, expecting to feel heat and it is quite cool, the burning is not due to raised temperature, but it may be due to the irritating sodium compound, NaOH (caustic soda), at work.
3. A burning pain arising when a motion is passed at the back passage is probably due to an excess of caustic soda in the moisture of the bowels, which may not be observed inside the bowels, but burns when passing the sensitive anus.

4. Anaemia.
5. Tiring unusually easily.
6. Excessive intake of salt.
7. Sciatica.
8. An abnormal blueness (indicating a degree of alkalinity) of the red litmus paper when pressed against the patient's moist gum under the top lip. Also when the urine and bowel evacuation are tested by red litmus. This is especially noticeable when only one member of the family is affected with cancer, and they all try the litmus test. They are impressed with the difference between the results of the patient's test and their own.
9. An extra alkalinity of the patient's blood as reported from the medical laboratory.
10. Constipation or inefficient action of the bowels and increased quantity of flatus (wind). If the cancer is inside the bowel there are often short attacks of diarrhoea with blood and mucus.
11. A weak pulse, not increased in rate. This appears to be a very constant sign in cancer patients; which is not surprising when one considers how the sodium robs the muscle cells of calcium, so weakening them.
12. Tetany, which is spasm of certain muscles, and painful cramp of the hands or feet or calves of the legs, especially as the patient is about to fall asleep. The facial nerves are extra irritable to tapping by the doctor with his finger tips. These conditions go with an increased alkalinity of the blood and a depletion of calcium. I have noticed some tetany of muscles in nearly all my cancer patients.
13. Frequent alkalinity of the urine is noted in a cancer patient when tested with red litmus paper.

The litmus may even show navy blue in the urine, although, on the same patient's gum test, the litmus paper may only show a pale blue colour reaction. This indicates that the chemical reaction of the body varies in different parts of the body.

CHAPTER VIII

A SIMPLE EXPLANATION OF HOW CANCER STARTS

When the particles of an irritating poison come into contact with, say, the mouth of a little sweat gland, the muscles of the sweat gland, if healthy, will contract violently and prevent the poison particles from lodging there. But, if the muscles of the sweat gland lack calcium, they are too flabby to contract and to squeeze out the poison particles. *We must realize that our body always seeks to protect itself, in every way it can, from injury.* Therefore, the appropriate nerve centre in the brain (an *involuntary* one) sends an order to the little cell (in contact with the poison) to multiply, and to do so quickly, and thus prevent the wretched poison particles getting into the body. The cells do multiply and they form a little wart-like structure, which is an act of protection.

We have discussed in earlier pages the method by which these cells divide and multiply, i.e. by the post-birth slower rate, when the irritating poison is limited in quantity and in the period of its application, and so the wart grows relatively slowly and is limited in size. It is classified as a simple lump; you might call it a surface adenoma.

The irritating poison that causes a cancer lump to form must be strong and continuously produced from the lymphatic channels, or in the blood-stream, to ooze out into the space around the body cells. The moisture around the cells circulates along the lymphatics, and back eventually to the heart. This is, indeed, what happens when there is an excess of sodium, and compounds of carbonate of soda, in our blood-stream.

There is now one very important thing to note, and that is that the compounds of carbonate of soda, in the blood-stream, do not have such a tendency to ooze through the walls of the blood-vessels into the surrounding tissue where that tissue is *soft,* and therefore forms no impediment to the contraction of the blood-vessels or the quick flow of blood in the blood-vessels, as in the *small* bowel. But, where the blood-vessels pass through some old damaged spot which has been repaired, chiefly with connective tissue, which is not elastic, it tends to impede and slow down involuntary contraction of the blood-vessels and therefore slows the flow of blood. This gives time for the more solid particles in the blood-vessels (i.e. the carbonates of soda molecules) to ooze out on to that spot. Some of the sodium carbonates are very unstable substances, and so they break up and liberate pure sodium which joins with any moisture present to form caustic soda.

The protective mechanism of the body is not idle at this time. The involuntary brain centre, governing the body cells nearest to the caustic soda, instantly orders them to multiply and multiply quickly at the pre-birth (much quicker) rate, and produce sufficient of the protective lactic acid to neutralize the soda and so stop harm being done. The irritating caustic soda loves acids most of all, and so it at once joins with the newly formed lactic acid, to form a neutral salt, a harmless lactate, which is washed away in the lymphatic stream.

Why Tumours Form
But, unfortunately, when more and more carbonates of

soda ooze out of the blood-stream at the spot, and more caustic soda is formed, then more and more of the cells in that spot multiply (to form protective lactic acid), and so the newly formed body cells eventually form a lump, which is called a tumour. Thus is a typical cancer tumour formed by our body to protect us from the burning caustic soda. The type of cancer tumour formed varies according to where the tumour first started. All secondary tumours in a patient are of the same type of cells as those of the first tumour. This is called *Nature's Economy of Effort*.

It seems apparent that either *one* involuntary nerve centre in the brain governs *all* the body cells of the same shape, or that the different nerve centres governing the same shape body cells are closely in touch (through their nerve fibre endings) with all the other nerve centres governing the body cells of the same shape. Some body cells are naturally much quicker growing than others.

Another potential site of cancer tumours is where the thin walls of the tiny blood-vessels are, for instance, on the surface of a mucous membrane lining a cavity. Excessive sodium carbonates in the blood-vessels are apt to ooze out of the thin walls of the tiny vessels on to the surface of the cavity. There they split up and give off carbon dioxide gas; soda is liberated and quickly forms caustic soda which does its deadly work on the surface of the membrane. Such cancer tumours may be formed on the inside of the lips, tongue, fauces, tonsil, gullet, stomach or big bowel. When in the bowel or stomach there is constant flatus (wind) formed of carbon dioxide gas.

My own personal experience, some years ago, of the agonizing pain of caustic soda being formed in my own body, and the heavenly relief afforded by the application of a dilute solution of hydrochloric acid, convinced me absolutely of the truth of Doctor Smalpage's contention in his book *Cancer — Its Cause, Prevention and Cure* (now out of print), that it is caused by the alkali, caustic soda, being formed in the body, and that it could be relieved by weak solutions of dilute hydrochloric acid. Doctor Smalpage also added tiny doses of phosphoric acid, in very special pills, containing one-fiftieth of a grain of phosphorus.

To emphasize the fact that secondary tumours consist of the same shaped cells as the primary, and that this is an economy of effort of Nature, I again call your attention to the fact that, when there is an involuntary order from the brain to, say, the eyelid, to flick to protect the eye from a sudden movement unpleasantly close, the ordinary person does not, at the same moment, involuntarily contract his arm or leg.

As sodium can be so dangerous it would seem to be better if we could try to banish it altogether; but, in its *right* quantity, it is as important to our well-being as air or water. Another peculiarity of sodium is that its proper function is in the liquids of the body. It preserves the correct density of the moisture of our body, and this enables nourishing particles to be received by our body cells, and their waste particles to be taken away. Whereas, the job of the elements *other than sodium* is concerned with the actual make-up of our various body-cell substances.

It is only when there is a great excess of sodium in our body, *and we are run down in health,* that we fail to neutralize properly and eliminate the excess of sodium. Then, as you have learned, it pushes its way into some of the body cells and turns out some of the other alkaline elements. This is particularly bad when one of the alkaline elements happens to be calcium, for, as I have said, if the muscles lose their correct quota of calcium, they become flabby and weak. This can be very bad when our heart muscles are concerned, as it is not hard to imagine. Therefore, excessive sodium can also play a part in the biggest cause of death — heart disease. This factor is, of course, more pronounced when the person does not take enough daily physical exercise, and eats excessively of pappy, non-stimulating food, such as white bread and other starchy foods, deficient in the necessary amount of natural minerals and vitamins which abound in whole foods and in green salads and raw fruits.

CHAPTER IX

HOW PRE-CANCEROUS WEAK SPOTS ARE PRODUCED

I feel it is most necessary that I should give a more detailed account of the factors liable to produce a weak spot in our body, thus providing a potential site for caustic soda to do its deadly work. I do this so that the cancer-producing process is understood thoroughly. We may now take it for granted that caustic soda is the continually acting cause of cancer in 99 per cent of cases of cancer.

The primary factors of degeneration producing a *Weak Spot,* may be:

I. *Physical,* such as mechanical irritants, contusion, a blow and friction, such as continuous rubbing.

II. *Thermal Agents.* These are abuse of heat through the medium of fire, electricity, boiling water, hot and cold beverages, ice cream, etc. Burning of the skin, as in some Asiatic customs.

III. *Rays* — X-rays or Radium, which break up harmless compounds of sodium, and thus cause the formation of NaOH (caustic soda). Solar rays may also cause excessive sodium carbonates to turn to caustic soda, as evidenced in cases of skin cancer developed on Sydney bathing beaches.

IV. *Chemical Agents* — Harmful chemical agents are innumerable, e.g. coal tar, tobacco tar, strong alkalies, such as potassium, also calcium (in quicklime), strong alcohol, various strong salts, hydrocarbons, etc., and many drugs.

V. *Bacterial Infections* — Previous bacterial infection, which has been overcome, but which has left a weak or injured spot in the body.

Irritants and irritations produced by the factors mentioned above, are encountered very often in daily life. When the body tissue is *normal* it has a natural resistance, and so the body cells degenerated by the primary irritant are rapidly regenerated to become normal cells, or replaced by normal cells; therefore the organism cannot become sick.

It is very important that we should have a clear knowledge of the foregoing facts, because there is a tendency by some superficial thinkers to blame one of the primary factors, which produces only a weak spot, and could never produce cancer without the presence of excessive sodium in that organism; be it bird, or animal, or human being. Fowls given much table salt in their mash often develop internal tumours, and sometimes an ulcerating tumour is to be seen, especially on the bare skin under a wing. Tumours inside the bodies of the fowls are often noticed when the carcases are being cleaned for market.

Excessive Sodium Treated Successfully

As an instance of how external poisons may cause a weak spot in the body, I will relate one of the many cases successfully treated by the methods I am describing in this book. This patient, a Mrs. W., was discharged from a public hospital about eight years ago, with a hopeless and inoperable disease of the pancreas. (The pancreas is a vital digestive organ close to the stomach, and it acts on the food that comes from the stomach.) This lady was very fond of strong pepper and hot condiments on and in her food. I have no doubt that these irritated the pancreas and set up a chronic inflammation of the organ. She also had an excess of sodium in her system (such a common condition!). She was a farmer's wife, and had lived the usual active life on a farm. Nothing untoward so far as her health was concerned had happened for years.

Her balancing internal mechanism had enabled her to neutralize and eliminate her excessive sodium; but her chemical laboratories had been working overtime to do so. Naturally, she was blissfully unconscious of anything being wrong. Then, when she became older — over 50 — pain developed rather suddenly, it seemed, in the region of her pancreas. Her internal laboratories had gone on strike, or had failed to act efficiently, due no doubt to tiredness or a run-down condition.

Bouts of pain became so agonizing that she demanded, and was given, various pain-killing medicines. When she was sent home from the hospital to die, as too weak to be operated on, her home physician was bidden watch her die, and dole out to her the pain-killers — the various nerve-numbing drugs.

At this time a relative of hers bade her go to me for advice and treatment. She lived over fifty miles away; but her husband motored her in to see me every week, although I wanted her to stay at least two weeks handy to my consulting rooms, so that I could instruct her thoroughly in the vital routine of treatment. I put her on treatment similar to that described in Chapter XIX to free her of excessive sodium, and check the disease. This treatment she carried out herself at home. Her recuperation at first was up and down, then she gave in, and came to stay nearer to me, with a daughter-in-law, who proved an ideal nurse, and invalid cook. In two weeks more, she was marvellously improved, and free of pain. She returned to her home to continue her good progress. She recovered and today is active, happy and very pleased. But her pancreas did not fully recover from the damage the caustic soda had caused it.

You will remember that I said the pancreas is an important digestive organ. This patient tended afterwards to have a little indigestion sometimes, as shown by flatulence (i.e., wind) but continuous doses of pancreas extract tablets remedied that. Five years later this lady developed a suspicious soreness and redness of her tongue. She came to consult me, and admitted she had been eating salt butter again, and using a *very little* table salt in her cooking. After some chlorine medicine and the stopping of table salt her tongue became normal again and she resumed her previous good health.

An important sign should be noted in human cancer, and that is the tumour's rate of growth, and the factors governing the rate of growth. Where the rate of growth is steadily progressing, there must be something in the body of a continuously progressing, irritant nature. Note that the human victim is daily continuing to take into his body an excess of sodium, in one form or another, in one food or another. It seems past belief that any educated person can believe that any part of the human body can suddenly grow, at the rate a cancer tumour often does, and then decay without rhyme or reason, yet that is the attitude some medical men profess to take.

CHAPTER X

CANCER OF THE LUNGS

Doctor Smalpage, in company with other eminent scientists, has commented on the great increase in the habit of cigarette smoking, which so often causes cancer of the lungs, by its irritation of the delicate tissues of the lungs and respiratory tract. He seems to infer that people inhale sodium in the use of tobacco. One thing is quite certain, however, and that is that nicotine is an irritant and that it produces little patches of inflammation in the lungs. This is proved by the chronic little cough of many cigarette smokers. We know that where there is an excess of sodium in the body, there is consequently an excess of the unstable carbonates of soda in the blood. It is well known that cancer often starts in an old injured spot; but what is not sufficiently widely realized is that some of the unstable carbonates of soda in the blood, when in great excess, ooze out of the blood-vessels into the tissues, and there disintegrate, where the sodium unites with some of the moisture and forms caustic soda. This settles on the nicotine-damaged spots in the lungs, cauterizes them, and forms cancer lumps.

Cancer of the lungs is a particularly painful disease and a fatal one. It is not curable by any methods used at present by the medical profession. I have known cases of cancer of the lungs to be helped towards recovery by methods which free the system of excessive sodium and build up the vitality. Of course, it is absolutely essential that there should be good co-operation on the part of the patient and his attendant, if he is fortunate enough to have a good one. I call the attendant my guarantor. A sick person is so apt to be forgetful, and sometimes careless. *Perhaps in no disease more than cancer is recovery dependent on good co-operation between attendant and patient.* I would rather have a case of cancer of the lungs to treat than cancer of the stomach, because the latter type makes the control of diet most difficult.

Some time ago I attended a medical meeting. One of the doctors there related an account of a medical experiment or, rather, an investigation, which had been concluded in Great Britain. Two and a half years before, over two thousand doctors were contacted, and they were divided into three groups (1) heavy smokers, (2) light smokers, (3) non-smokers. After two years they were again investigated. Some of the heavy smokers were dead of cancer of the lungs. Some were suffering from cancer of the lungs. Of the light smokers none was dead, but some of them had cancer of the lungs. Of the non-smokers none was dead and none had cancer of the lungs. When the doctor had finished relating this account there was silence for a few moments, then one doctor remarked that he did not hear so many matches as usual being struck!

CHAPTER XI

SOME IMPORTANT COMMENTS ON CANCER

When you are trying to eliminate excessive sodium, during the first two months of treatment, one should, of course, *not partake of sodium in anything.* It is a good thing to precede treatment by spending two days on nothing but fluids. Take frequent drinks of warm water to which a dessertspoon dose of Stock Vinegar, that is, *chlorine water* (see page 102), is added.

Even if one is sceptical about dietary treatment, it is obvious that it can do no harm. Sufferers will usually be delighted at the relief from severe pain even by the end of only the third week, and that often without anaesthetic drugs. Frequent hot baths give some patients relief. There is a form of cancer where there is not so much pain, because the tumour is impeding local circulation by pressing on blood-vessels, causing an exudation of fluid, which presses on the nerves, numbing them.

There are many types of cancer, depending entirely on what group of body cells is affected. Some cells multiply much more quickly than others. Cancer characterized by a type of cell which grows especially quickly is called sarcoma, and it is especially malignant.

The present stupid treatment of cancer is merely to cut out the lump — if this can be done without the patient dying on the operating table. Even if the patient dies next day, the surgeon will still claim that the operation was a success; but he often adds, 'It was the patient's fault he died; he should have come earlier for treatment.' This is a constant and grim joke to medical students. No effort is made by the surgeon or his doctor to find the *irritant* cause of the tumour formation.

(a) Radium a Painful Treatment

An effort should always be made *first* to find the cause of the irritation, and to remove it, before operating. Because, if the irritant cause of the tumour remains, the tumour will only be repeated, sooner or later, after the operation. This constantly happens. If, however, the tumour cannot be removed by surgery, then X-rays or radium are used. Radium burns, and by breaking up sodium carbonates in the part treated allows the sodium to promptly form sodium hydrate (caustic soda). This burns the affected part and causes occlusion of the blood-vessels there, preventing any fresh sodium being brought to the part, and so the tumour in that spot is checked. But it is, usually, a very painful treatment. Of course, this form of treatment can only be carried out if the tumour is on or near the surface of the body.

(b) X-rays Can Prove Fatal

If X-rays are used, they do not have any effect, of themselves, on the actual cancer cells, but they cause the sodium carbonates, *elsewhere than in the tumour,* to disintegrate and form caustic soda. This may relieve the actual tumour for a time, but the patient feels dreadfully ill, and as if he were burning all over, which, of course, he is, with caustic soda forming all through him. He feels very sick, and is red in the face, and he sometimes vomits repeatedly. The patient's tissues are burnt all over him, and uric acid is formed, with which the sodium promptly joins to form a sodium urate; and these urates are washed away in the urine. If you examine the patient's urine before the treatment, you will not find any urates of the uric acid sodium type in the urine; but, after the administration of X-rays, you will find the patient's urine loaded with them.

One cancer patient I was treating said to me, 'I had one treatment of X-rays a month ago, and it made me feel terribly ill. I am just getting over it, and now the hospital has sent me a message that I have to come up for a second treatment by X-rays. Shall I go or not? I dread it!' This was when I also had consulting rooms in the City of Christchurch. She used to come up to my rooms nearly every day. Not knowing as much about the X-rays treatment then, as I do now, I said to her, 'I suppose they know what they are doing. Perhaps you had better go.' The result was that she became progressively worse, and she could no longer call at my consulting rooms. I had to visit her. She had been progressing wonderfully well under dietetic treatment; but after the second treatment of X-rays she became so deteriorated in health that I could not rally her at all, and she gradually died.

Can you blame me that I have never sent a cancer patient for X-ray treatment since? And I have never sent a cancer patient to be treated by surgery; because I know surgery cannot cure cancer. But I have sometimes advised surgery to remedy some injury to the body done by the burning caustic; or by the blockage of some important tube or duct by the tumour, or to remove adhesions.

Where a colostomy has been advisable, I have always begged that it would always be of a *temporary* nature, so that when the cancer tumour, blocking the alimentary canal, was dispersed, the natural opening of the bowels at the back passage could be restored.

No surgeon can guarantee in writing that operative treatment has permanently cured his patient, or that the tumour will never return. This must be so, because he tackles only an effect, and ignores the cause of the tumour formation. Therefore, the surgeon generally bids the patient to report to him for an examination every three months, to see if he has got a return of the tumour; which, of course, can be expected when the cause of the tumour has not been removed.

Now, cancer is not infectious, nor is it inherited; but you can inherit a tendency to a weak liver or weak kidneys, and so have a lowered ability to cope with any excess of sodium. Also habits of eating and cooking are often passed on from one generation to another.

The ordinary patient with cancer becomes progressively and visibly ill. He loses weight, loses energy, becomes weaker and very anaemic, and very sallow-looking, especially at the last. He is lacking in the vital supply of oxygen. Bouts of severe pain set in, and as the disease advances, even the strongest anaesthetic drugs do not completely relieve the severe pain, or for only a short period.

Cancer Can be Stopped

Cancer is truly a terrible and cruel disease. It can be prevented — it can be stopped. Just because the secondary lumps always consist of the same shaped cells as the primary lumps, medical men ignore any influence the involuntary brain centres may have had on the body cells, and so come to the erroneous conclusion that the so-called secondary tumours arise from the direct spreading of infection, as it were, from the affected cells of the first growth that took on the abnormal rate of growth.

I repeat the following for emphasis and to help understanding.

There is no doubt that every particular sort of shaped

cell in our body has undoubtedly got its own centre in the brain. If some alkaline irritant over-stimulates one sort of body cell, these particular cells send a message by their own particular nerve fibres up to their own particular nerve centre in the brain (like the involuntary flick of your eyelid at some near movement in front) and back comes the order, through the involuntary nerves, 'Multiply quickly, ever so quickly at pre-birth rate.' Any of the cells of that particular shape, anywhere else in the body, may be affected, and take on quick growth, and form tumours.

It is known that the sodium neutralizer, lactic acid, is given off by the cells when multiplying. Some of the lactic acid unites with the alkaline caustic soda (NaOH), and so forms a neutral, harmless substance, sodium lactate, which is carried around in the lymphatics to the heart, then through the blood-vessels to the kidneys and excreted in the urine. If, however, the patient is run down in health, the sodium lactate is not excreted by the kidneys in sufficient amount and so lumps are formed. The nerves acting in these cases are what are called nerves of the sympathetic system. Therefore, the lumps, called tumours, are really an effort of Nature to protect the body from the burning caustic (NaOH).

The lumps do not kill the patient unless they are pressing on a very vital spot. What often kills the patient is that some of the caustic soda burns into the little blood-vessels, and the cancer patient may finally bleed to death. It may be internal and, therefore, hidden; but there is often a statement, by the nurse, that blood came away in quantities near the end of the patient's life. The patient may die of lack of oxygen through severe anaemia. Certainly in some bad cases of cancer, near the end of the patient's life, it is said that quite a number of different shaped cells take on *rapid* growth and form tumours all over the body.

Irritant Poison

Much depends on the amount of sodium, and the ability of the body to cope with it. It has been found, by experimenting in a vivisection laboratory, that various irritant poisons continually applied to one spot on an animal's body will produce a tumour, of a cancer type.

In the case of a wart, which is caused by a similar reflex action from the brain, the poison comes from the outside of the body, and the wart does not grow very much, because the irritant poison is limited in duration and quantity. In the case of a cancer, the poison comes from *inside* the body and the protecting growth has to increase in bulk to do its protecting work; because the cauterizing caustic soda is continually and increasingly being formed and bombarding the lump. This often causes some of the newly formed cells to break down and ulcerate and discharge and bleed.

The *first* thing that happens in the case of the cancer tumour is that the patient is overcharged with unstable carbonates of sodium in his blood-vessels. That is the result, no doubt, of his internal balancing, neutralizing, and eliminating laboratories working overtime for many years; but he has been of course, quite unaware that anything serious was amiss.

Then the patient becomes run down in health, through *breaking* continually one or more of the Ten Commandments of Good Health (read carefully Chapter XVIII). It may be due to insufficient sleep and wrong diet, or not sufficient suitable outdoor exercise, or inefficient action of the bowels, or a combination of all. In addition, he may possess a weak or injured spot on the surface of, or inside, the body, which provides a starting place for a cancer tumour.

Such a spot may result from:

1. A physical cause, such as a blow.
2. Some old bacterial action, as from an old, infected milk duct in the case of a woman.
3. Some chemical poison.
4. A previous burn, or from one of many other injurious causes as I have indicated in Chapter IX.

Cancer of the Breast

Cancer growth in a woman's breast is very common, because the breast has no big, quickly flowing arterial blood supply; but it has a great number of rather small blood-vessels, and the blood in those does not circulate so quickly as if they were big arterial vessels. Also in the breast there is a mass of lymphatic vessels. Tight brassieres, or a heavy, pendulous breast, may also add to the slowing of the circulation. These conditions give the carbonate of soda particles the opportunity to ooze through the blood-vessels on to an injured, and thus sensitive, spot, and there form caustic soda, with the consequent rapid multiplication of cells, and the start of the cancer process, if the person is run-down in health.

Milk is always exuding from the milk ducts in the nipples. It is true that it is in very tiny quantities when a woman is not pregnant, indeed, in so tiny an amount that a woman is generally totally unaware of its presence. Milk is one of the finest cultures in which bacteria can flourish, and so the milk ducts may be infected by bacteria, if the nipples are not very carefully guarded by keeping them extra clean. If a nipple does become infected, the infection may spread up one of the lacteal ducts and form spots of inflammation, and so a thickening or a lump in that area may be noted. Nothing more may happen, but if the woman becomes run-down in health, and her blood is overcharged with the unstable carbonates of soda, some may ooze out of the slower-flowing blood-vessels on to the deteriorated spot. Then the carbonate of soda is split up and sodium is liberated. We know that sodium will never stay by itself for a second; and so if there is no protective acid present, it immediately joins with two-thirds of a molecule of water to form caustic soda. *This so irritates the body cells in that spot that they at once start to multiply.* Sometimes, the multiplication is, at first, at the comparatively slow post-birth rate. This liberates the protective lactic acid, which neutralizes the caustic soda and so she is protected for a longer or shorter time from the formation of a quick-growing cancer tumour. Further, she may, in all probability, have enough vitality to eliminate the sodium compounds, and so she may never develop a cancer tumour; she may only have what is called a simple tumour or adenoma.

However, if later she should deteriorate in health and her vitality become too low to eliminate the sodium lactate compounds quickly enough, an increasing amount of sodium carbonate will ooze on to the deteriorated spot, and more and more caustic soda will then be formed. Then the body cells there will multiply more speedily at the *pre*-birth rate. The process goes on, although the cells, by multiplying increasingly quickly, neutralize some of the caustic soda, but more is continually formed in that spot, and so the cells multiply even faster than at pre-birth rate. Many of the cells do not even stop to form properly, and the caustic soda cauterizes many of the cells in the tumour, with the result that it ulcerates and bleeds. She now has cancer of the breast. There is a continuous stabbing or burning pain, from which the patient generally demands any form of relief. The pain-killing drugs that are usually administered not only do not cure : they actually render the patient worse, by hampering still further the work of the internal vitalizing laboratories.

The breast is one of the least difficult places to treat for cancer, because unlike the digestive organs, it does not provide any obstacle to the exceedingly necessary diet revisions for cancer patients.

Other Forms of Cancer
In some cases of cancer, an operation will sometimes prove helpful, in order to give time to free the patient of excessive sodium, such as when the cancer is in the big bowel, and it has caused a blockage. Then a *temporary* colostomy may be helpful as I have said elsewhere, so that dietetic and other treatment can reduce and remove the excessive sodium. In cases where the common duct from the pancreas and gall bladder is blocked, in cancer of the pancreas, a union of the gall bladder to the intestines is necessary. This operation is more likely to be successful if the effusion in the patient's body is first drained, and in such a case a blood transfusion may help. The common duct I have referred to is that which conducts juice from both the liver and the pancreas to the intestine. In such a blockage the patient would be very jaundiced.

In several cases of cancer of the pancreas with which I have had to deal, there was a history that the patient had been very fond of pungent food, e.g. pepper, mustard, and chillies. I have no doubt that the pancreas had been first weakened through the continual irritation of the products of such items.

In cancer of the oesophagus (gullet), when it blocks the passage of food to the stomach, a temporary tube fixed into the stomach enables one to more easily nourish the patient.

When the cancer is in the bowel, and the patient suffers

a burning pain when passing a motion from the back passage, an enema of dilute hydrochloric acid, in the dilution of one teaspoonful of dilute acid to 1½ pints of warm water, gives wonderful and instantaneous relief. He may be so tender at the back passage that he can only stand half a pint at a time; so give several successive half-pints of the fluid, as may be tolerated.

There is one thing which the cancer patient, or his attendant, should bear in mind, and it is that even if at the first they do not have great faith in the methods I have described, they must realize, that at the very least, the treatment will do no harm. If they will painstakingly carry out the technique of treatment, they will be delighted beyond measure with the result.

Importance of a Vegetarian Diet

Some cancer patients do not see, at first, why they should adopt a vegetarian diet; but if they read this book carefully they will surely see why. Where the cancer has affected the liver it is especially important that they keep strictly to a vegetarian diet, until such time as *their vitality is fully restored, which may take up to two years of strict perseverance.* Of course, the excess in alkalinity, and the growth of the cancer tumour, may be stopped in seven or eight weeks, in the *average* case of cancer. But if an important organ or part has been destroyed by injudicious operation, or radium, or X-rays, or if the presence of a great excess of sodium, with very poor vitality, is causing leukaemia, one may not be able to save the patient's life; but he can be given ease, and his life may be prolonged when nothing else is of avail.

Do you remember that our blood contains two main classes of cells? There are millions of little red cells whose function is the bringing of oxygen *from* the lungs, and the taking of carbon dioxide *to* the lungs. Then there are some slightly larger cells called leucocytes and these are less in number in the blood. They are generally globular in shape, somewhat similar to the little red cells, but they have the power of movement, of temporarily altering their shape, and they are light in colour. The wonderful thing about them is that they seize any foreign matter, such as dead tissue or microbes, and ingest them, and so try to destroy them. They act as a sort of scavenger. They are sometimes spoken of as our policemen. Scientists call them phagocytes, and their power of engulfing and digesting foreign particles is known as phagocytosis.

I have explained before how dependent we are on the work of the little red cells in the blood, and of their procuring oxygen for all our little body cells. They take the carbon dioxide (CO_2) from our body cells and carry it in the blood-vessels to our lungs, where they exchange it for oxygen, which they bring back to our cells.

We may be compared to a slow combustion engine. Therefore like all things that burn, we must have oxygen. Our cells need oxygen to produce heat, energy and body substance. In the healthy body this process goes on without interruption; but when we are charged with excessive sodium there is an interference with the smooth running of this cycle. When the stomach seizes the chlorine out of the sodium chloride particle, the bereft sodium may seize a carbon dioxide particle, forming a carbonate of sodium, which seems to travel round in the blood quite harmlessly.

Now, as long as there is sufficient carbon dioxide for both the processes to continue in a balanced manner, i.e. for the taking of carbon dioxide from the body cells by the sodium, and also enough for the little red cells to take to the lungs to exchange for oxygen, nothing amiss may occur. In these circumstances there may be a little excess of sodium occasionally, creating an extra alkalinity of the blood, but without having sufficient vitality to cope with it, no trouble ensues. However, with further and continued unbalance, a *simple* tumour may occur.

Appetizing Food

It is essential that the average cancer patient should not lose any more weight, especially if he or she has already lost a good deal. Food should be made appetizing and dainty, but there should be plenty of it, especially in the first serving. Never ask patients what they will have, or if they will have a second serving. Just bring it in, and very often, the patient will eat it all. Whereas if you asked him he would likely refuse it.

Although acids and starches at the same time can cause indigestion, as evidenced by flatulence and wind, so much depends on the relative quantities. Take a helping of stewed fruit directly after having eaten potatoes, and you invite wind and indigestion. But a tiny tomato, or a slice of tomato, eaten with the potatoes, will not be harmful, if it is just enough to give a relish. Again, potatoes with a green salad that has previously had an acid dressing poured over it, would be all right if you avoid too much of the acid liquid. You will know by the results. A slice of rich plum cake, that has been made without raising powder, would not harm the cancer patient. Jam on bread and butter would not be harmful, if it is not ladled on. A dozen or more raisins, just covered with water, and boiled one minute, and then spread on bread and butter, are good.

CHAPTER XII

DISEASES CAUSED BY EXCESSIVE SALT

We must remember at all times that a total of a quarter of a teaspoonful of table salt is a sufficient amount for the twenty-four hours, *from all sources*. Some biochemists say that a level teaspoonful is a good average per twenty-four hours. In any case, the average person takes many teaspoonsful in the butter, bread, bacon, fish, cooked vegetables, confectionery, beer, etc., etc., he takes during any one day. Added to these sources is sodium bicarbonate which has been substituted, in our modern baking-powder, for ammonium bicarbonate, which our grandmothers wisely used. Excessive sodium can produce at least twenty different diseases, of which cancer is one. These occur when the body is so run down in health, from constantly breaking one or more of the Commandments of Good Health, that the body cannot continue to cope as it has done with the excess.

A LIST OF SOME OF THE DISEASES THAT CAN BE
CAUSED BY EXCESSIVE SODIUM :

Constipation, more rarely dysentery.

Heart disease. Various anaemias, and leukaemia.

Lowered resistance to various infections. Thus, excessive salt may be a contributing factor to influenza, tuberculosis, infantile paralysis (poliomyelitis).

Various cysts, as of the thyroid, the ovary or the uterus. Hydrocele. Stones in the gall-bladder, the kidney or the urinary bladder.

Asthma, nasal septum troubles, nasal catarrh, polypoid growths, rhinitis sicca, polypoid rhinitis, frontal sinusitis, mastoid inflammation; fibroids, disseminated sclerosis, adenoma, ulceration of the uterus, oedema, migraine, rheumatism (which is also produced by excessive acidity of the body). Ulcers, skin troubles, and various eczemas, itching, burning, or weeping skin, cramps, and tetany. (This last trouble, tetany, I have observed in one form of another, at one period or another, in nearly all my cancer patients. It is an involuntary twitching or cramp of some muscle; and it can be very painful. It often occurs at night when falling asleep.)

Sodium the Irritant Cause of Cancer

The above list of diseases is given in his book by Doctor Smalpage, of Sydney. He found out in his laboratory that excess of sodium was the irritant cause of cancer, in a debilitated constitution; and that cancer can only be cured by first getting rid of the excess of sodium in the body. Doubtless, he has seen and treated all the diseases listed above; but I have met only some of them since I learned that excessive sodium was the irritant cause of cancer. Those I have met and treated made such a good response to my anti-sodium treatment that I am convinced that Doctor Smalpage is correct in all the statements that I have quoted.

Now, I test every patient who comes to my consulting rooms to see if they have an excess of alkalinity in their blood, which constitutes alkalosis. Sometimes they come to me and say that they are suffering from acidity, i.e. acidosis. And I surprise them, and sometimes myself, in finding out (per the litmus paper test) that they are suffering from the opposite condition, namely alkalosis. It is wonderful how quickly they benefit when I put them on to an anti-alkaline regime; and how pleased they are at the improvement in their health. Of course, some of these patients are not so run down in health as to have developed cancer; and so it is easier to benefit them. But such patients are potential cancer victims.

Always remember we can dig our graves with our teeth, and that we can help build up longevity and good health by eating only the right food; we can be a credit to our community by always endeavouring to keep all the rules of good health, and those in regard to eating, especially. Maintain the correct balance between the alkaline and acid elements as explained fully elsewhere in this book.

Migraine, heart trouble, and cancer I have experienced myself as a result of excessive sodium intake, and being at the same time very run-down in health and over-worked. But, knowing the cause, I cured myself. I have helped many cancer patients by neutralizing and ridding their bodies of the excessive sodium, and putting them on a good, wholesome *salt-free diet* making it *strictly vegetarian,* for three months, and as much longer as the patient cares. The vegetarian diet can be made delicious and very stimulating with its natural vitamins in its raw salads. It is wonderful how quickly the patients' pain goes and they start to improve. But they must, at the same time, carefully observe all the *Laws of Good Health* which I will describe in detail in Chapter XVIII. I have often found it most difficult to make patients realize how very important are all these laws. Good results depend greatly on the *careful co-operation* of the patient and his attendant in carrying out the laws of good health.

CHAPTER XIII

WHAT YOU SHOULD KNOW ABOUT YOUR FOOD AND DRINK

Class I — Water

Water is very important. Many people do not take enough plain water each day. We should not take less than one and a half pints of liquid per day, as water, fruit juice or as it is in the food we eat. It is not good to take much liquid at a meal, as it is apt to dilute, and so weaken, the digestive juices. It is a good thing to take drinks mid-morning and mid-afternoon, or at least an hour before or one or two hours after meals. Nothing should be eaten between meals, with the exception of fruit.

Class II — The Carbohydrate Foods

Group I — *Starch*. This is predominant in wheat flour, and grains (cereals). The universal practice of milling wheat and discarding the germ and husk, merely leaving concentrated starch, cannot be too greatly condemned. The resultant greatly impoverished flour is used in a multiplicity of confections, cakes, biscuits, etc., etc., by almost everybody. Many vegetables, notably potatoes, beans, peas, and legumes of all kinds, contain starch.

Group II — *Sugar*. The sugary foods are cane sugar, and all things made with it, treacle, golden syrup, etc. The best source of sugar is honey, and the sugar present in the various foods, as grape sugar, lactose, maltose and glucose.

Group III — *Fats and Oils*. These are butter, cream, the fat of meat, nut butter, oil as found in various seeds and nuts. Pure cotton-seed oil, peanut oil, sunflower-seed oil, soya-bean oil, etc., and the oils of certain fish, such as cod liver oil and halibut oil.

Class III — The Protein Foods

Group I — Animal proteins include all meats, such as beef, mutton, pork, veal, bacon, ham, fish, poultry, and all things made from them. Other protein foods are cheese and eggs, as well as concentrated skimmed milk powder.

Animal proteins leave more ash, as uric acid, in the system. This is the basis of many diseases, if not properly eliminated.

Group II — Vegetable proteins, e.g. peas, beans, lentils, split peas, and pea flour. These vegetables also contain starch and so they are included under that heading as well. Soya bean flour is especially valuable as a protein because its starch content is insignificant. The germ of wheat, present in good wholewheat bread, is also a good protein.

Nuts in their great variety. Pine kernels and cashew nuts are very good, as is salt-free peanut butter, sold by many health food shops. Then we have desiccated coconut, chestnuts and chestnut flour, and gluten meal. Some include gelatine, jellies, and isinglass in this list, although their protein content is quite low. Protein foods are very important in replacing tissue waste; but so many people do not realize that very much less is needed after we stop growing, and still less after middle age. If taken in excess the carbohydrate foods and the animal proteins tend to be organic-acid-producing. Never forget that quantity is as important as quality!

Class IV — The Cleansing Foods

These are vegetables and fruits, raw, with their 'life' and their vitamins and minerals. We should always take some raw food at least at two meals per day : if it is only raw onion, or parsley, or mint. Vegetables always contain more vitamins and other valuable nutrients before cooking. Raw spring onions, tomatoes, apples, lemons, and cress are especially rich in vitamins needed by the body. All grated raw vegetables and raw green vegetables are especially good. Vitamins may be said to oil the wheels which make life go round, and are, therefore, vital. No food can be properly assimilated and used by the body without its *own* vitamin or vitamins. It is pitiful how much food is literally wasted because it is eaten without its own particular vitamin content, lost in its manufacture or cooking.

Class V — The Mineral Salts

The chief ones are salts of iron, magnesium, calcium, sodium, potassium, manganese, and copper. These are the chief *alkaline* inorganic elements : then there are the salts of *acid-forming* inorganic elements, such as iodine, chlorine, phosphorus, and sulphur. It is vital to our health that we should have a daily sufficiency of these substances, and in the *correct proportions*. These elements are largely supplied in the vital vegetables and fruit. They diffuse into the water they are cooked in, therefore it is exceedingly stupid to throw away any water in which vegetables have been cooked. Vegetables should be cooked conservatively, so that their natural flavour, vitamins and minerals are retained as far as possible. Any liquid used for cooking vegetables should be saved to drink or for use in soups, gravies, etc.

CHAPTER XIV

THE IMPORTANCE OF CORRECT DIET

I personally had to start to study the food I ate before the age of ten years, in order to overcome my frequent bilious attacks which were accompanied by severe headaches and distressing palpitation. These troubles were overcome by the time I was thirteen years old, when I was permitted to go to school. I have had to diet ever since! The useful thing has been that I have very frequently found that foods good for myself are also good and curative for my patients. I have had some marvellous cures as a result, especially remarkable in patients who have been sent home from a public hospital to die as hopeless cases. Patients who have had all the usual bad methods of drugs, knife and X-rays, and have been given up as hopeless, have made seemingly miraculous recoveries under the good hygienic treatment and good diet I have put them on.

The history of tuberculosis seems to have taught medical men nothing. It is a well-known, and an acknowledged fact, that drugs and operations will never cure tuberculosis without the appropriate good diet and good hygiene.

There is no black magic in dietetic treatment. I only do what any other doctor could do, if he took the trouble to teach the patient to live according to the laws of good health. The word 'doctor' means 'a teacher.' In this book I am trying to state all the practical details of the successful treatment and cure of disease so that any intelligent person can apply them. Of course, a man with medical training could do wonders, if he so chooses, with the information I am endeavouring to make clear. *But* these three things *must* be applied simultaneously : first and foremost, *diet;* second, *hygiene,* and third, *medicine.*

As I have said before, acid formation in our body, apart from in the stomach, is bad, and so is excessive alkalinity. We must try to maintain in our body fluid a balanced reaction of very slight alkalinity. Please understand that the word *slight* is very important; i.e. *quantity is as important as quality.* Take one laxative pill and you benefit; but if you take a whole boxful at once you will suffer. Most people have suffered from a bilious attack through eating excessively of some rich food at one meal; whereas if they had taken only a small amount no harm would have ensued.

Milk is Not a Drink

Reverting to the fact that quantity is as important as quality, a good instance of this is seen in milk. A great many people take pure milk as a drink, when it should be taken only as a food; and so in this way they take more nutriment than the body can deal with. As a result, a lot of mucus is created, and then we have catarrhal conditions. If you are always spitting up mucus when you have not got a cold, cut off, or cut down on, your milk ration, and you will be surprised to note how much the mucus will be reduced. A well-known food specialist said that drinking milk not only causes mucus, but it often causes inflammation of the mucus glands and lymphatics, and is the chief cause of tonsillitis in children. If, instead of cutting out the tonsils, the milk ration of the child was cut down, a most marked improvement would be noticed in inflamed tonsils. Personally, I think it would do school-children more good if they were given a nice clean apple to eat at school, instead of the drink of milk. Children should be taught the necessity of washing fruit, even before peeling, because of the possibility of thread-worm eggs in the dust on fruit skins, and because the results of fruit sprays need to be washed off.

CHAPTER XV

SOME GENERAL OBSERVATIONS ON FOOD ELEMENTS

To cook conservatively, grease (mind *only* grease) the bottom of the pot with fat or oil, and put in the vegetables and place the pot over an element turned to top heat; then add a cup of hot water, and at once turn down the heat to the lowest point. The food will cook nearly as quickly as food with a lot of water cooked on the hottest element. Prolonged high heat destroys vitamins. If you are a good and careful cook you will never burn your vegetables. In certain cases, one may have to add tablespoonfuls of water from time to time. And, of course, one must dish up vegetables as soon as they are cooked.

There should be no difficulty in getting children to eat vegetables conservatively cooked. They are delicious; and quite different in taste from those that are overcooked and drowned in liquid so that their flavour and vitamins are lost in the steam, and their minerals dissipated in the water. No wonder baby refuses to eat such food until he has been made to acquire the vicious taste for table salt that is added to make the 'murdered' vegetables palatable. Even the man of the family cannot tolerate the usual badly cooked vegetables until he has sprinkled them with table salt, or the cook has done so. I say that they taste like wet blotting paper! Thus is laid daily, in unneeded table salt, the seeds of at least twenty different diseases, of which cancer is one. Note, too, that the mineral salts of vegetables, as well as those of fruits, are vital to our blood and the various compounds of our body.

Always remember that sodium is one of the most dangerous elements when taken in excess. Table salt and soda, put into the water vegetables are cooked in, destroy much of the valuable vitamins. Vitamin C is destroyed completely. Therefore, always cook vegetables so that they do not lose so much of their good minerals and vitamins. Properly cooked vegetables are especially essential to the cancer patient. His body has shown a weakness in dealing effectively with excessive sodium. He should therefore be careful for the rest of his life.

While I am on the subject of the effect on health of what goes into the mouth, I would like to say that I am whole-heartedly with those doctors who condemn the fluoridation of our public water supply. If it is going to be in sufficient strength to affect medically one section of the community, it will certainly affect everyone; and it will affect some to their harm.

It is certainly not going to help the children's teeth while they are being rotted with an excess of Class II food, such as white bread, cane sugar, sweets, pappy food and so on. Fluorine will never supply the minerals and vitamins of Class IV and Class V foods (see Chapter XIII). These foods are not luxuries but necessities for children's health and good teeth. For every pound that governments might spend in subsidies to make such valuable foods available to all, it would save the taxpayers more than a thousand pounds for the cost of disease — drugs, doctors, hospitals, and the like. It is said that the children are a nation's greatest treasure. Well, study the physique of the school-children of any government school as they march in their hundreds. Many children are of shocking posture. Chins are the most advanced part of their bodies; they have curved backs, they stoop forward with hollow chests, and they have pale faces. People newly arrived in New Zealand from Britain often comment, with surprise, on the children's pale faces. Listen to them playing! Too often you hear not the happy cries of children at play, but hysterical shrieks . . . One wonders how far the cinema is responsible. In Austria, before World War I, Austrian nerve specialists got the government to forbid children under twelve admission to picture theatres. Surely something is wrong, when, in this lovely country of New Zealand, we are said to have the highest percentage of lunacy of any English-speaking country.

You may say to me, 'What have all the foregoing remarks to do with cancer?' The answer is, 'A lot,' because all things that lower vitality make the individual less able to cope with excessive sodium in his body.

Fluoridation Increases Cancer

This chapter would not be complete without some further reference to the evils of water fluoridation. Fluorosis is what the *British Medical Journal* called the evil result, in an article that starts with the heading, 'Absorption of Fluorine Compounds causes Chronic Poisoning.' It goes on to recite many of the very evil effects fluorine compounds have on our body, and it quotes nine scientific authorities in support of its condemnation.

Then elsewhere I read a statement by Madame Louise, of Australia, that a huge American aluminium manufacturing company have a large by-product of dangerous sodium fluoride. They were trying to persuade various nations to use it in their public water supplies; and it was stated that they were offering money to various public authorities to propagate it as being good for children's teeth. They were getting one and a half cents a pound for their by-product as rat poison; but when they sold it for human consumption they got many times that sum.

It is admitted that more than one part per million of
sodium fluoride in our drinking water is not potentially
poisonous. But food cooked in such water would contain
much greater and, therefore, potentially poisonous
amounts. This is doubtless one of the reasons that more
than 800 cities and towns in the U.S.A. have either
rejected or discontinued fluoridation of their public water
supplies. When a New Zealand public-spirited man, a Mr.
Robinson, offered a cheque for £1,000 to anyone who
could prove that any public water supply under fluoridation could always be kept within the safe margin of one
part of sodium fluoride per million of water, no one
accepted the cheque. Which demonstrates very clearly that
fluoridation is an ugly menace. Even if it were good for the
children's teeth, it is destructive to adults' teeth. This fact
is demonstrated in photos in the *British Medical Journal* of
December 10th, 1955.

There is no doubt that fluoridation of our public water
supply would very much increase cancer; because of the
impossibility of avoiding excess of sodium in such a water
supply. Sodium fluoride accumulates in the body, and it is
only when it reaches a certain amount in the body that it
suddenly shows its poisonous effect. Note that sodium
fluoride often causes great pain in the joints of old people.
Fluorine has a great thirst for calcium. There are two sorts
of compounds of fluorine :

(1) The organic forms, as found in Nature, always
contain some calcium.

(2) The inorganic forms, when introduced to our body,
at once seize some of its calcium content, such as that of
our muscles, weakening them. This is especially injurious
when our heart muscles are robbed of calcium. The trouble
is that the organic forms (that is, the natural forms of
fluorine compounds) are not very soluble, whereas the

inorganic forms, such as the dangerous sodium fluoride, are very soluble.

Surely there must be sufficient of the natural calcium-containing organic forms of fluorine in New Zealand for the people's teeth, judging by the splendid teeth the Maoris had before the Europeans came to New Zealand with their health- and teeth-destroying foods.

A very sober thought — *under fluoridation it will become impossible to cure cancer,* because we will not be able to rid the cancer patient's body of excessive sodium by diet, when his drinking water contains sodium, as well as so much of his food.

CHAPTER XVI

WHAT RADIATION AND X-RAYS DO
FOR CANCER

The present favourite method of cancer treatment with most doctors is to have the tumour cut out, if this can be done without killing the patient on the operating table. Alternative methods of treatment are through the medium of radium or X-ray applications. These have no effect on the cancer cell itself; they only affect the mineral compound, the carbonates of soda, which are present and which they break up, thus liberating the atoms of sodium. Now, if there is no acid present for the sodium to join with, it promptly unites with the nearest water moisture and forms caustic soda compound (NaOH), which acts on the body cells nearest it, cauterizing them, and causing agonizing burning pain.

Consider the apparent success, sometimes, of radium implanted on the surface of the body tissues for treating cancer near the surface. What happens? Any effect of the radium is entirely due to the radium breaking up the sodium carbonates in the tissue fluids, and changing them into caustic soda. This action here is slow. The effect of the slow formation of caustic soda causes fibrosis (thickening and contraction) by tissue destruction, thus cutting off the blood supply to the tumour. This leads to the atrophy of the tumour, also to the slow breaking up of the sodium carbonates in the tissues surrounding the growth, before their caustic product can touch the actual tumour. This removes the main cause of the tumour increasing in size by the multiplying of its cells to form the protective lactic acid. Without the cause, i.e. the irritating caustic soda, the cancer tumour cells must undergo disuse atrophy. This disuse atrophy may be exceedingly slow, years maybe. But radium implanted thus is very painful. Dr. Smalpage explains this very clearly in his book.

X-rays have no effect on body cells nor on cancer cells; but they do affect mineral compounds. If we want an X-ray picture of the inside, say, of the stomach or bowel, we have to fill it first with some mineral substance, through the medium of what is known as a bismuth meal, which patients dread because it is heavy and uncomfortable. They have to take a laxative afterwards to drive it out; and if there is a tender ulcerated spot anywhere this is irritated, and feels sore after the bismuth meal has been purged out. The patient may declare he feels worse, and he probably is!

Of course, the meal is given only for the purpose of the X-ray examination, to enable the doctor to see clearly what is the precise condition.

Lung Cancer from Cigarettes

There was a case I came across some years ago, of a woman, elderly and feeble, with gastric ulcer of eight years' standing, which her doctor considered had now turned to cancer. She had signs of cancer of the lungs. She had been a cigarette smoker for many years, and she had burning pains across the top of her chest, and pain on breathing. The bouts of pain in the stomach due to the gastric ulcer increased in severity. Also she had a burning pain sometimes in the left lower side of her chest, just above the waist line. Her attending doctor said she was too feeble, anyway, for an operation, and that she was a hopeless case of cancer, quite incurable; but he wanted to give her a bismuth meal and have her X-rayed. But she and her attendant nurse-daughter refused. Then he said he would not see her again until she agreed, and that meant that she would have to go without the pain-killing drugs he had been prescribing. As I have just said, he had previously informed the daughter that her mother was a perfectly hopeless case.

However, this patient improved wonderfully when she adopted proper dietetic treatment, and she is still alive after eight years, free from pain without drugs, and able to go for little walks.

Doubtful Benefits of X-Rays

Now, to return to our consideration of X-rays. Cancer growths are ray-sensitive purely and simply because the sodium carbonates present are converted by the X-rays into caustic soda. The degree of so-called radiation sensitivity is entirely dependent on the degree of saturation of the tissue fluid with sodium carbonates. The smaller the amount of sodium carbonates present, the smaller the degree of radiation sensitivity. This essential sodium carbonate factor for radiation and for effects on tissues from the use of radium or X-rays, discloses why many clinical symptoms and pathological conditions arise as the result of these radiations on cancer patients.

What happens in cancer depends chiefly on the quantity of sodium and the degree of vitality of the body to deal with it. Consider that in *deep* X-rays, the cancer patient, after exposure, has varying degrees of nausea, vomiting, physical and mental prostration and a sensation as if the body is on fire. What produces these constitutional symptoms? Let me repeat that X-rays convert the sodium carbonates circulating (away from the tumour) in the cancer victim's blood and body tissue fluids into sodium hydrate (caustic soda) and so the body tissues are burnt. The protein substance of the body cells is burnt, and destruction occurs. Uric acid is formed, and this combines with the caustic soda to form the mild sodium urates.

To prove this, examine the patient's urine before treatment with X-rays, and no urates will be found in it. But after the treatment the patient's urine is loaded with urates. This undoubtedly removes the burning and irritating sodium from the site of the tumour for a period, but any permanent benefit is doubtful. *Too often the final result is death.* I have observed this personally in patients so treated by other doctors.

Eminent Doctors Condemn Surgery
Let us now discuss surgery for curative treatment. Read carefully Chapter XVII. It quotes from statements made by many eminent doctors who are opposed to surgery as a cure for cancer. They say it not only does not cure, but very often it makes the patient worse. Admittedly surgery is sometimes necessary, temporarily, to remove or alleviate the damage the caustic soda has done to some part of the body, or when the tumour blocks some important tube. Many eminent doctors not only condemn surgery as a cure for cancer — but they also condemn burning with radium or X-rays, which is just stupidly treating *one patch of the body* for cancer, when the *whole body and system* is affected and untreated.

Many doctors entirely ignore the controlling action of the involuntary centres in the brain. So many eminent doctors have condemned the present surgical and radiation methods of treating cancer that it is almost incredible the way it is persisted in by the rank and file of medical men. Is it because their vanity will not allow them to admit that they were wrong? Or, as some hard critics suggest, the reason is that the financial returns are good under the present system.

I thought it very fine of Sir Stanford Cade, an eminent surgeon of London, who visited New Zealand towards the end of 1955, when he told a big meeting of medical men here, in Christchurch, N.Z., that he no longer believed in removing a woman's breast for cancer. He said he had seen 25,000 breasts removed for cancer; and that in every case, sooner or later, the cancer returned generally in a more inoperable place in the body. He said he did not know the cause of cancer. He mentioned that there were a quarter of a million people affected with cancer in Great Britain. And he said he believed it was rapidly increasing in the Commonwealth. After he had flown back to England it was reported in the *Star-Sun* (an evening paper of Christchurch, New Zealand), on December 14th, 1955, on the cable page, that Sir Stanford Cade had given a lecture to the Royal College of Surgeons, in Manchester, England, in which he said 'that inoperable cancer was no longer incurable, and that modern discoveries in chemotherapy (that is medicines) can bring the patient into the same line of diseases as diabetes and other constitutional diseases. He said advances in the efficient management of inoperable cancer are the result of a clearer understanding of the disease, and the natural history of the disease, and application of rapidly developing knowledge. He also said that cancer could be brought into other groups of diseases.

I would like to say that I had presented Sir Stanford Cade with a copy of Dr. Smalpage's book on cancer, and said that I had proved many times that Dr. Smalpage was right in his statement that the cause of cancer is sodium excess. I do not know how far that influenced him in the statements he made when he arrived back in England.

In spite of what Sir Stanford Cade said, not the slightest

impression seemed to have been made on the majority of the medical men here in New Zealand. They have gone on operating on cancer patients the same as before.

CHAPTER XVII

DOCTORS' VIEWS ON SURGERY AND RADIATION FOR CANCER

Many doctors in England oppose surgery as a cure for cancer; and some of them say that surgery not only does not cure, but it makes the patient worse.

Dr. Stanton, of Sydney, who was Registrar of a large hospital there, said, at a medical conference on cancer, that only 5 per cent of those operated on for cancer were alive after five years. He said he thought that any other method of treatment than surgery, or X-ray, or radium, should be thoroughly investigated. Yet the medical fraternity in New Zealand and the health authorities in New Zealand often refuse to consider any other methods.

A doctor well known in England, Dr. L. Duncan Bulklay, said, 'Cancer is not cured by the knife. It is no more reasonable to consider cancer a local disease to be cured merely by surgery, X-rays, radium, etc., than it would be to try and cure gout, rickets, syphilis or tuberculosis merely by treating a local symptom and ignoring the constitution. We must first seek what is wrong with the patient's system and try to rectify it by proper constitutional measures. By so doing many of us have cured cancer without the knife, which is so rightly feared by the people.'

Dr. Weedon Cooke, for twenty years surgeon to the Cancer Hospital, London, made a very similar statement; as did also Professor Syme and Sir Benjamin Brodie, who is a world-renowned doctor.

Also Dr. R. Mallett said, 'The knife is a delusive hope. It merely terrifies, and poor wretches are mutilated. If they survive, and are not warned to reform their bad habits of feeding . . . Nature will eventually revolt, and cause further development of the cancer disease.'

The late Lord Horder, a physician to the British Royal Family, said he believed that the crude method of merely cutting out a cancerous growth is not a cure in the true sense.

Diet Reform Can Avert Cancer

Dr. F. W. Alexander, Medical Officer of Health for Poplar, London, said, 'Nothing but a reform in our habits of eating and drinking and smoking and medicine taking can avert the death march of cancer, which is killing twice as many people as it did ten years ago. Cancer seems to be hereditary in some families, only because wrongful methods of cooking and eating and living are perpetuated in such families.'

Dr. T. Barker points out how bread is robbed of its important vitamins and is often bleached, and such chemical ingredients added as are dangerous to the people's health. Animals fed on it die. Whereas if fed on wholemeal bread they flourish. Many doctors who have lived amongst natives who live on natural foods say these natives never have cancer. But when they change their diet for ordinary American or British diet, they become prone to develop cancer.

Sir Robert McCarrison stated this also in the American *Medical Times*, and Dr. Veitch, who worked among the Polynesians and Melanesians said the same. So did Dr. William McGregor who practised medicine in British Guiana for over nine years. And Dr. Johnson (who practised in Lagos on the West Coast of Africa for fourteen years) also corroborated this.

Dr. Hislop and Dr. Fenwick, of New Zealand, say cancer is on a rapid increase in New Zealand, where the people are hearty eaters of meat and white bread and regular tea drinkers and tobacco smokers, and that nothing, to date, is done about it.

According to some insurance companies' statistics of 1954, there were fifty-five people dying every week of cancer in New Zealand, i.e. roughly over 2,800 people per year. That is a greater percentage, in comparison to the population, than in Great Britain, where a quarter of a million people were affected with cancer. Of these, 16,300 died of cancer of the lung and respiratory system. And 261 children under five years of age died of cancer in Great Britain. But to continue with important references.

Haliburton's standard work on physiology, used in many medical schools, points out that the mineral salts, especially calcium and sodium, are important in correct amounts and in correct proportion to each other for the proper action of the heart; and that an alkalosis, due to excess sodium, causes a lessening of the tonic calcium in the blood, which has a weakening effect on the heart by depriving it of the very vital calcium. Such an effect also happens to the muscles of the intestines and is largely responsible for chronic constipation.

Dr. Estes, of Chicago, says the ancients warned people against excess sodium, as seen in carvings on stone tablets.

He says, 'Excess sodium can cause oedema, also loss of hair, hardening of the arteries and impaired vision, defective hearing, dizziness and insomnia, and extreme sensibility to pain, also undue irritability of the nerves, melancholia, bad habits, perversion and unbalance of our mineral content.'

He said he thought fifteen grains of table salt, i.e. about

a quarter teaspoon, was the proper quota from all sources; that is the amount that should not be exceeded per twenty-four hours.

Those great doctors of biochemistry, Cameron and Gilmour, lecturers in biochemistry at a Canadian university, think that sixty grains of table salt per day from all sources is a good quantity for the average adult but they also say that people take great excess of this to their detriment. Everyone should read their book, *The Biochemistry of Medicine* (Publishers, Churchill, London).

As long ago as 1902, Dr. James Braithwaite, M.D., held that common salt was cancer causing. Then in 1906 Dr. Shaw Mackenzie, in his well-known book, *The Nature and Treatment of Cancer,* said that all his cancer patients used salt excessively. Since then hundreds of doctors have made the same observation. E. D. Robinson, M.D., of the National Biochemical Laboratory, Mount Vernon, New York, has described sodium chloride (common salt) as 'the most active cancer cause among inorganic agents.' Other doctors, like Dr. Haig, speak of salt as a contributory cause of cancer. An expert research worker in biochemistry, Dr. R. Keller, D.Sc., of Basle, revealed that many of the leading personalities in Eastern Europe adopted a low salt diet. Patients at a famous sanatorium near Dresden, and some fifty other sanatoria, are for the most part kept on a diet which is low in sodium chloride (common salt) and rich in potassium as found in raw vegetable salads and raw fruit. Dr. Gerson treated growths in this way in New York hospitals. In some cases, for a period, even the sodium normally present in the food is eliminated from the diet. This enables the potassium and other important salts in the body to become active where previously their normal function was interfered with by the excess of sodium chloride.

It has been pointed out that in the closing years of the nineteenth century there was a high cancer mortality in Japan where people lived largely on salted fish. It was not until the consumption of this salted fish had been materially reduced that this cancer scourge was reduced.

In 1946 *Cancer* (an official publication of the American Cancer Society) published a twenty-page report by five prominent medical research workers stating that 'X-rays (also gamma-rays) may cause cancer of the bone [which is a very painful form of cancer]. Thus there is conclusive evidence that X-rays and radium have no place in the treatment of cancer. They represent another attempt to deal with symptoms rather than causes of disease. They weaken the body, sap the resistance and may hasten death if too much is given. Many cancer patients die of the excessive treatment with X-rays, radium or surgery. Their deaths can be attributed to functional or anatomical deformities produced by these treatments.'

Now please note the following : The famous and great surgeon of the Mayo Clinic, Dr. C. H. Mayo, says, in the *American Medical Journal,* Vol. 2, page 213, 'taking a biopsy [extracting a tiny bit of the cancer tumour] often aggravates and stimulates the malignant growth — and does not indicate how many secondary tumours have developed.' Yet, in New Zealand, every surgeon orders a biopsy of nearly every one of his cancer patients; especially if he sees them in the early stage of the disease. Thirty years ago Dr. G. Everett Field, Director of the Radium Institute of New York, observed, 'blindly we have been attacking cancer in the advanced stages for many generations with surgical efforts, only to find prompt recurrence after removal.'

In 1946, Dr. Herman J. Miller, world-renowned scientist and Nobel prize winner, warned a Senate Committee in the

U.S.A., 'that there is no dosage of X-rays so low as to be without risk of producing harmful spreading of cancer to other parts.'

The Lancet, of November 12th, 1938, stated, 'Cancer often resulted in other parts of the body as a result of a local application of radium.'

Cancer is a Blood Disease

The eminent Dr. Robert Bell in the New York *Medical Research Record,* March, 1922, said, 'Cancer is a blood disease and must be treated as such. For seventeen years I operated on my cancer patients; but then I became certain that cancer is a constitutional disease, and is both preventable and curable by *proper diet,* and by *building up* the constitution. So I gave up the most lucrative part of my practice (i.e. surgery for cancer). I noted that during those years of my surgical practice that in spite of the fact that operation treatment for cancer was being performed by the tens of thousands, the cancer death rate had gone up 200 per cent.' When he was Head of the Battersea Hospital, England, he said, 'Surgery and X-rays are ineffective to cure cancer.'

Dr. W. A. Dewey, a Professor of Medicine at the University of Michigan, wrote, 'In a practice of forty-five years I have yet to see a single case of cancer, save a few semi-malignant epitheliomata (skin cancer), cured by surgery, X-rays or radium.'

Dr. E. C. Folkman, editor of *Scientific Therapy* and a practical research worker, said, 'When as a physician I had seen the terrible destruction and sloughing of the whole half of a patient's face some months after the application of radium needles, I decided never again will I recommend the use of radium. The remedy is worse than the disease.'

Dr. O. Theron Clagett, famous Mayo Clinic surgeon, said

on March 1st, 1955, 'Radical surgery is not the answer to cancer, because the knife fails to remove all possible routes of spreading' — he said he was certain that eventually cancer would be cured by medicine.

Cancer is Not an Isolated Happening

Dr. Nikolai Blokhin, of the Soviet Academy of Science, declared in 1954, at a Cancer Congress, that 'as a result of a long series of experiments, we know the cancer tumour is not an isolated happening; but an illness of the whole body. Soviet scientists consider cancer is due to a number of agents, including chemical and physical factors, which may bring about alteration in the metabolism, and in certain conditions provoke cancer. A long series of experiments have shown that the growth of the tumour depends on the general health of the body.'

Now, it is very important that while the excess of sodium depletes the body of other alkaline elements, it is not safe to try to replace them whilst the reaction of the body is excessively alkaline. It is necessary first to reduce the excessive alkalinity before any attempt is made to replace the other important alkaline elements such as calcium, potassium, iron, and magnesium. It will be noted in Chapter XIX, that I was careful to take no oranges in the first month, and not more than one a day in the second month. This is because oranges are particularly rich in potassium. After the second month, the oranges would help indeed to reduce the excess of sodium if taken in moderation. Prunes, tomatoes and swedes are in the same category as oranges.

Only a comparative few of the doctors who have publicly condemned operation, radium, and X-rays, as a cure for cancer have been named. There are many more doctors who have said the same. Several of my references to the statements of eminent medical men condemning surgery, radium, and X-rays as a treatment for cancer, I have quoted from H. M. Hoxsey's book, *You Don't Have to Die* (Keystone Publishers Inc., New York). I think it was also in this book that an important American doctor referred to the disgraceful practice of some doctors in regard to the procedure of split fees. This means that if a physician sends a patient to a surgeon for operation, the surgeon gives the physician a slice of the fee he gets for the operation.

Sir Robert McCarrison, of the British Army Medical Service, on duty at a post in the Himalayas, said 'that in the nine years he was there he had not treated any native for cancer, appendicitis, gastric or duodenal ulcer, gallstones, colitis, rheumatism, or any of the usual pests of civilization. The natives were restricted by religious dogma and poverty to the outgrowth of the ground for food, with the exception of milk and cheese, of which these people used but little, their chief diet being vegetables, fruits, nuts, and whole-grain breads.' McCarrison says that the older men of the tribe looked so much like the younger men that he was often not able to tell the one from the other as they worked in the fields. They reported great ages; the older men were so efficient that they took their part in wrestling and other strenuous sports.

Dr. W. H. Hay said in his book, *A New Health Era*, that 'we could keep well if we would quit making ourselves sick; and also if we ate less meat, white flour, and cane sugar, we would escape the danger of autotoxicosis [self-poisoning].' He reminds us that the important thing to remember always in our food is the value of it for digestion, absorption, and its utilization by the body for heat, energy, and body substances. Our ability to eliminate the ashes (waste) in the system should be kept at a high level. He is very emphatic that we should note the chemistry of foods, by which we should realize the danger of combining acids and starch at the same meal among other things. Both are good if taken by themselves, but often quarrel when taken together, as is often done when a plate of stewed fruit is taken with a milk pudding.

CHAPTER XVIII

THE TEN COMMANDMENTS OF HEALTH

The following Ten Commandments of Good Health must be obeyed by all who have developed a chronic disease. *It is imperative that they are followed most conscientiously and persistently. Half measures will be of no avail, therefore there should be no compromise.*

I.   Thou shalt have sufficient Fresh Air (no chilling).

II. Thou shalt have sufficient Warmth (no cold feet, no blue legs in winter).

III. Thou shalt have sufficient water (inside and outside).

IV. Thou shalt have sufficient Sunshine (not on the tumour).

V.   Thou shalt have sufficient Sleep (eight hours in bed, minimum).

VI. Thou shalt have sufficient Exercise (daily walks out of doors, the best).

VII. Thou shalt have sufficient Relaxation (fully reclined).

VIII. Thou shalt have sufficient Elimination (per bowels, skin, kidneys, and lungs).

IX. Thou shalt have sufficient Cheerful Attitude.

X.   Thou shalt have sufficient Balanced Food.

Food Must Be Right In:

    (a)   Quality.

    (b)   Quantity.

    (c)   Time of eating (regular five-hour intervals).

    (d)   Rate of eating.

(e) Proportions. (No big slabs of meat with a minute helping of vegetables, and so on. Don't eat all protein and no starch, and vice-versa.)

(f) Combination. (Acids and starches at the same time do not agree, especially with cancer patients.)

(g) The mental atmosphere in which it is eaten.

REMEMBER IN CONSIDERING THE FOREGOING COMMANDMENTS OF NATURE THAT SHE IS VERY KIND WHEN OBEYED : BUT HARD AS STEEL WHEN DISOBEYED. OBEY AND LIVE — DISOBEY AND DIE.

Let us now elaborate on the Ten Commandments of Health.

I. We must have pure air containing sufficient oxygen, without any poisonous fumes. While it is good to have open windows, it is not good to sleep in a *draught* that chills, which sometimes happens by having the door open as well. (Some tubercular patients have developed a fatal pneumonia through their attendants overlooking this.)

II. *Warmth.* Cancer patients generally feel the cold, because their circulation is poor, and so they must be especially guarded against getting chilled. Their feet must be kept warm night and day. Cancer patients will benefit if they are kept in the fresh air as much as possible. An easy chair, rugs and a cushion, and perhaps a hot-water bottle. may help to make possible staying out of doors. The part affected with cancer is often eased at first with cold packs, and later by hot packs. Apply whichever gives the most relief.

III. *Water.* Water is best taken, as a rule, about blood heat, and about an hour before or an hour after a meal. Midway between meals is good. It is all right to take a few sips of fluid with meals; but there should never be taken so much fluid that it over-dilutes the digestive juices, and so produces indigestion. Unless the food taken has much moisture in it, not less than a pint and a half of water should be drunk in the twenty-four hours. Two pints are good. Water is so purifying. Of course, if your food is dry you need more water. But the exact quantity depends on the size of the individual, his work, and the climate.

IV. *Sunshine.* Avoid sunburn; but be in the sunshine whenever possible, at least for a short period. The sun should not be allowed to shine on any cancer tumour, as it may induce any sodium carbonates present there to form sodium hydrate, which is caustic soda (NaOH). Sunshine does not induce skin cancer unless there is an excess of sodium in that person. Indeed, if there is no excess, sunlight is more likely to help to prevent cancer, as anything health-promoting does. One will have a good idea if there is likely to be an excess of sodium in the system by considering one's dietetic habits, and the result of the red litmus paper test per gum and urine. Also, a burning sensation at the anus on passing faeces indicates the presence of excessive sodium.

V. *Sleep. Note well:* nothing from a chemist's shop can take the place of sufficient natural sleep. Never less than eight hours *in bed* is advisable for a worker, if he wants to live out his span of life. If one cannot sleep, one must relax. It is best not to read in bed. Sleeping tablets are bad — very bad. They are all so unnecessary. To promote sleep take more daily exercise in the fresh air. Walking exercise is good, but do not undertake any exercise likely to cause haemorrhage in any cancerous condition. Some people cannot take meat, fish, eggs, cheese, at the last meal of the day, and sleep well afterwards. Such people should have cooked vegetables, with unsalted butter, or a salad, including onions and parsley, with a sweet, if desired.

VI. *Exercise.* It is essential for everyone to take each day a certain amount of active physical exercise. This is preferably taken in the form of walking, as briskly as possible, for distances depending upon one's vitality and ability. If possible, as much as a mile or two at one stretch would be excellent. In these days of motor transport people are becoming less and less inclined to convey their bodies through the medium of their own motors, their muscles. Never forget that *Life is Movement* and *that which stagnates dies.* These are immutable laws of Nature.

Where it is not possible to take walking exercise, recourse should be had to the regular daily practice of exercise movements. Breathing exercises that, when practised regularly and conscientiously, increase one's ability to take in oxygen — a vital need in cancer subjects — should be taken daily.

EVERY DAY ONE SHOULD, IF AT ALL POSSIBLE, ALSO PRACTISE SELF-MASSAGE, AS FOLLOWS :

Press firmly on the muscles of one arm with the opposite hand, as if to press the contents of the arm upwards towards the heart. Repeat this with the other arm, and then on one leg and then the other. Always go upwards towards the heart — this stimulates the circulation. When doing this to the lower limbs, you can use both hands for the pressing on each leg.

In any case of cancer, care should be taken that any contemplated exercise would not be likely to cause a haemorrhage.

VII. *Relaxation.* Relaxation is very important. It is necessary that everyone should relax sometimes during the working day, and not be keyed up all the time. When you feel tension rising, lie down for a period of rest. Some people relax by changing their work for a while; others find it more restful to lie flat on their backs, and try to think of nothing in particular. This last plan is very good. Taking stimulants such as tea, coffee or alcohol, keeps a number of people over-tensed all the time. They are never properly relaxed. This weakens their nerves. According to one well-known nerve specialist, more women in Great Britain went into the mental hospitals through excessive tea drinking than any other cause.

The alkaloid drugs, theine and caffeine, in tea and coffee, respectively, whip up the nerves, and alas these same drugs, or another equally harmful, is the stimulant in the universal soft drinks. Need there be cause for wonder that in New Zealand, where even more tea is drunk that in Great Britain, they have the unenviable reputation of having more lunacy per 1,000 of the population than any other English-speaking country?

For those who desire a hot, refreshing drink, there are a number of various preparations, quite innocuous, that may be obtained from health food stores.

VIII. *Elimination.* We eliminate waste matter by the lungs, skin, kidneys, and bowels. Walking exercise out of doors and deep breathing are most helpful in this task of elimination, as well as in building good, healthy muscles everywhere; muscles with a good quota of calcium, and not flabby muscles which have been weakened by having been robbed of their calcium by excessive sodium in the system. This is the cause of more constipation of the bowels than any other thing, especially when combined with lack of out-of-doors exercise.

If you are obeying the Laws of Good Health, and taking proper exercise, your internal laboratories will eliminate through the skin inoffensive and non-irritating perspiration (sweat) to your benefit. On the other hand, many skin diseases are caused by irritating perspiration due to excessive sodium. Regarding the bowels, some scientists have stated that, if a person has a desire to pass a motion from the bowels, and does not do so, within twenty minutes the poison in the faeces will begin to be reabsorbed into the system of that person. This is, of course, especially disastrous to a sick or delicate person. One woman told me that she complained to a nurse that her husband had not had his bowels opened for four days, and the nurse had replied, 'Oh, that is nothing in this ward.'

IX. *A Cheerful Attitude.* One beauty queen said you could not be really beautiful unless you were good. God is always more willing to help than we are to ask or listen to Him. And this applies to good health as well as beauty. Cultivate an optimistic frame of mind. Have faith in yourself and what you are doing to build health. As you get better so will your cheerfulness increase.

X. *Balanced Food.* We require the correct foods to provide heat, energy, and body substance.

(a) They must be right in *Quality.*

(b) They must also be right in *Quantity.* There must be sufficient of the various sorts of food we need daily — proteins, carbohydrates, fats or oils, minerals, and vitamins. If we habitually eat more than we require, we overburden and wear out the digestive organs, and, especially, the eliminating organs. Most people have excessive appetites — mostly young folk, although some old folk eat more for the sake of being occupied and for social purposes. Such people should decide, before they begin a meal, on the limit to which they will go. Again, other people have no appetite until they have eaten a few mouthfuls. These people are probably overfed already and so the body has no desire for further food. They should examine their appetite (or lack of it) in the light of this possibility and act accordingly. A good book on dietetics should be purchased and studied well and its recommendations followed.

(c) *Time of eating.* It is important to have your three main meals at the same time every day. Your digestive organs have been conditioned by behaviour to be ready then. They are very punctual in their demand. If detained well beyond a meal time, it is generally better for one to abstain from solid food until the next meal time, and have instead of a meal a drink of milk, or cocoa, or milk and barley-water, or some ripe fruit juice. Avoid any drinks about whose origin and preparation you are doubtful. A dessertspoonful of the special Stock Vinegar (described in Chapter XIX) to a cup of hot water, makes a most beneficial drink in the early stages of treatment.

(d) *Rate of eating.* Bolting your food is asking for indigestion. Chew your food thoroughly, and never gobble it.

(e) *Proportions.* I have many times seen a thick slice of meat with a tiny helping of vegetables on a young person's plate. This is bad. It would be better to have, roughly, seven times the bulk of vegetables to one of meat. Burning condiments should be taken sparingly if at all. *They are best avoided by a cancer patient.* Hot condiments injure the pancreas and predispose to cancer. Excessive sweet-eating, especially taking too much devitalized white sugar, is bad. One patient of mine admitted taking seven cups of tea a day with two teaspoons of sugar in each cup — fourteen teaspoons in all! Small wonder he was a patient.

(f) *Combinations.* It is bad to take starchy food, such as potatoes or milk pudding, at the same meal as you take stewed fruit. Starches do not digest in the presence of an acid. Acid fruit is best taken three-quarters of an hour after a starchy meal. Of course, bland fruits, such as the various dried fruits like raisins, sultanas, and figs, or bananas, can be eaten without trouble at meals which include starchy foods. If you are strong, with a good digestion, you may not observe any strain on your digestive organs with unwarranted mixtures of foods. But if you are below par in health you will experience flatulence, or wind from fermentation, or, maybe, eructation, or a red nose (and so incur the suspicion that you are a drinker of alcohol which, perhaps, you never touch).

(g) *Mental atmosphere at meals.* Nothing, perhaps, interferes with digestion more than a mental or emotional upset at meals. I have known a cancer of the liver start as the result of years of a person being upset three times each day at meals. The habit of taking worries to the table is bad, and invites indigestion. Forget them for the time being, anyway, while you are eating and digesting your meals.

CHAPTER XIX

HOW I CURED MYSELF

What I am now going to outline is the comprehensive treatment regime which I followed on treating myself for cancer of the bowel. Reference to what I have said in the previous chapters will confirm that the treatment was directed, in all its aspects, towards normalizing the physiological functioning of the system, and thus reducing the cancerous condition and rebuilding my health.

I realized only too well that, if I were to succeed in curing myself it would be necessary to adhere *implicity* and *conscientiously* to a very strict health-building regime, and that *any deviations would have rendered the treatment unavailing.*

In dealing with any case of serious illness I have always tried to enlist the assistance of a person other than the patient to act as a *guarantor* that the instructions are carried out exactly. Patients frequently are not sufficiently resolute to keep undeviatingly on the narrow path of correct treatment. They feel that slight departures will not matter, particularly when they notice some improvement. A firm-minded guarantor to supervise treatment overcomes any weaknesses on the part of the patient, particularly as he or she (the guarantor) will have a wonderful objective in view — helping someone to regain life's greatest blessing — good health.

THE NATURAL CHEMICAL TREATMENT

In treating myself for cancer, I used the following

preparations of medicine (not drugs but natural chemicals) which I regarded as indispensable:

(1) The first medicine was *ammonium chloride* in seven and a half grain *tablets,* obtained from a pharmaceutical chemist. I took one tablet three times daily, half an hour after meals.

(2) *PINK MEDICINE BOTTLE.* This consisted of acid phosphoricum dilutum B.P. (liquid diluted phosphoric acid) and liquid extract of amaranth. The chemist was asked to make a mixture of acid phos. dil. in the proportion of ten drops to a drachm of water, to fill a pint bottle. This was tinted pink with extract of amaranth (a harmless vegetable extract) to identify it. This medicine has a *faint* acid smell. The dosage was a teaspoonful in two tablespoons of water half an hour after each of the three daily meals.

(3) *TINCTURE OF IODINE MIXTURE.* The chemist made this up in the proportion of one drachm of tincture of iodine to four ounces of water. (When not in use it was kept well corked.) *Dosage* was one teaspoon of the mixture *once* daily at any time. I continued to take this medicine even after recovery.

(4) *TRANSPARENT MEDICINE BOTTLE ('STOCK VINEGAR').* This was made up from standard strength acid hydrochloric dilutum, B.P., obtained from the chemist in a four ounce bottle.

(a) I made up a dilution of one tablespoon acid hydrochloric dilutum to half a pint of cold boiled water, and placed it in a clean glass bottle which I labelled 'Stock Vinegar.'

(b) Each day I prepared a second dilution from the acid hydrochloric dilutum as received from the chemist, and placed one teaspoonful of it in a pint and a quarter of cold boiled water, in a quart-size glass bottle which I labelled

'Acidulated Water.' In my opinion, it played a very important part in my recovery. I took half of the amount made (i.e. five-eighths of a pint) warm or cold, mid-morning, and the other half mid-afternoon. Freshly expressed carrot juice was added occasionally when a change of flavour was desired.

SPECIAL MEASURES DURING THE FIRST MONTH. A quarter-pint (no more) of milk was taken each twenty-four hours with a teaspoon of the Stock Vinegar added to it. I used a plastic spoon, because a metal one tended to stain badly from the acid if I forgot to rinse it immediately after use.

SECOND MONTH. The milk was increased to half a pint daily, acidulated with a dessertspoon of Stock Vinegar, although I did not regard it so essential to take the milk after the first month. However the *Acidulated Water* was always taken an hour before breakfast — half a pint diluted with 50 per cent carrot juice. (In the first two precious months the drink should not be taken later than 8 p.m.)

As a variant, a tablespoonful of Stock Vinegar, added to half a pint of carrot juice and pure water, was taken instead of Acidulated Water. I continued taking this drink after the end of the first two months, as I regarded it as very necessary for safety and progress.

I always use Stock Vinegar in place of ordinary vinegar, and always for salad dressing.

THIRD MONTH. I dissolved enough epsom salts to cover a new penny piece in a tablespoon or more of water and took it once daily. I continued to do this until normal regular bowel activity returned. When I was satisfied that I was free from excessive sodium, I took tablets of calcium gluconate, with vitamin D, twice a day for six months.

FIRST AID FOR PAIN

When a cancer patient is in great pain, I have found that, apart from an anodyne hypodermic, which must be given by a medical practitioner, it is a good thing to give a dose of sweet spirit of nitre, say half to one teaspoon in water, and give him plenty to drink of acidulated water ('Stock Vinegar') to help to neutralize the caustic soda, and to drain it off as far as possible via the kidneys. A hot bath is helpful, especially if the patient is sponged all over afterwards with hot water and dilute hydrochloric acid, a dessertspoon to the quart. Make the patient sweat, if possible. Give the patient six grain capsules of pulvis calcium chloride after meals, three times a day. Give him frequent drinks of warm barley-water containing, per pint, a dessertspoon of Glucose D, and a tablespoonful of 'Stock Vinegar.'

To get the bowels to act, I have found that enemas containing a teaspoonful of dilute hydrochloric acid to a pint and a half of warm water are good. If it is possible to reach the painful spot, apply warm water containing a teaspoon of diluted hydrochloric acid to a pint and a quarter of water, and this should give relief.

MY DIET FOR THE FIRST
THREE MONTHS

I had *NO* meat, fish, cheese, or white of egg during the first TWO months. The yolk only of one egg every second day, during the second month, when chemical tests proved good (i.e. the litmus tests) and also if the liver was acting well. Diet was strictly vegetarian for the first three months, and I continued to exclude meat as far as possible afterwards because vegetarian protein has less waste poison than animal protein.

NO fruit drinks containing preservatives.

NO cane sugar, or only a *very* limited amount.

NO tea, coffee, alcohol, or cola beverages.

NO condiments (pepper, mustard, cayenne or chillies).

NO nicotine — *NO* smoking.

NO table salt or anything containing it. The list of these foods is long, and so it was necessary to be *very* careful.

NO sodium in anything. Table salt is 50 per cent sodium. Commercial baking powder is full of sodium, so I had *nothing* with ordinary baking powder in it. *NO* sodium bicarbonate.

NO aspirin preparations of any kind.

NO borax. Butchers and fishmongers use compounds of sodium and often sulphate of sodium. Too often manufacturers use compounds of sodium to preserve dried fruit and lentils and dried peas, dried beans and split peas. Therefore, all these were soaked overnight and well rinsed; then they were placed in cold water and brought to the boil and then kept simmering until cooked. They were tested with red litmus paper for alkalinity, if I was at all doubtful.

NO acid fruit at vegetable meal (sweet fruits, such as raisins, sultanas, dates or figs are not acid fruits). When raisins or dates are used, I prefer to buy them *with* the stones in, wash them well and then take out the stones.

NO fruit preserved in sugar syrup. I ate only salt-free cereal foods such as salt-free porridge, or salt-free bread.

SPECIAL NOTES: All my butter is salt-free — a rule I shall follow all my life, to avoid a relapse.

N.B. Ordinary salt butter contains thirty grains — that is, half a teaspoon — of salt to the ounce. The amount a *healthy* person should eat of table salt should never exceed sixty grains (one teaspoon) per twenty-four hours, adding up *all* one gets from *all* sources.

NO oranges, grapefruit, tomatoes, dried fruit, or swedes, during *the first special month,* but I had these (oranges, once daily) for the *second* month. I always take a teaspoonful or more of wheat germ (*Bemax, Froment,* etc.) daily on some of my food.

Onions, chopped raw and sprinkled or mixed with cooked food, such as potatoes, give a relish and one does not then miss the table salt so much. Some of the juice of an onion may be used on cooked food for flavour. Powdered onions may also be used, where suitable, for added flavour. Grated or finely chopped raw green vegetables also add zest, and help one not to miss table salt.

N.B. Heat, if high, destroys the vitamins in foods. The value of vitamins consists in their enabling one to assimilate the substance in which they are present. Vitamins taken on their own, without their parent substance, act as acute stimulants at the moment, but they drain and sap the patient's vitality eventually, if persisted in.

BREAKFAST MEAL (Meal No. 1) *I was very careful to avoid any food which experience had shown to upset the liver.*

My breakfast consisted of fruit, especially raw fruit, nuts, *and after the third week,* a little milk, or half a cup of junket, or yoghourt (unsalted). Nuts were sometimes grated. Fresh fruit salad was a favourite dish.

Some raw fruit was always taken daily. Apples, well washed, were a favourite, taken grated sometimes.

N.B. Dried fruits, such as washed raisins, sultanas, currants, figs (soaked), and prunes (soaked) were not taken until after the first month of treatment; they have a relatively high content of organized sodium, which is valuable when a person is in health, but not when overcoming a condition caused by excessive sodium. The fruit meal was taken only at breakfast or mid-day, not in the evening.

Five or six dates were used in green salad, or in the dressing, to lessen the acid taste of the 'stock vinegar', after the *first* month. Occasionally, I had porridge (oatmeal, or wheatmeal) for breakfast (no salt) with some of the acidulated milk allowance, and a tablespoon of fresh, untreated cream on top of the porridge. (I made sure there was no borax or bicarbonate in the cream.) Half a teaspoonful of treacle, or golden syrup, or honey, was added for flavour, when desired. As an alternative, I had two or three slices of salt-free bread with salt-free butter, plain or toasted, with the butter spread cold, and with sultanas, or sliced onion, soaked dried fruit, ground nuts, or *ripe* bananas.

If the porridge seemed to disagree, sometimes I omitted the sweetening or had wheatmeal porridge instead of oatmeal. From three-quarters to one hour *after* the starchy (cereal) meal, I took fruit in plenty (I counted apples to be best); but bananas are good at any meal, cooked or raw.

I made it a rule that acid fruits, such as plums, peaches, gooseberries, fresh currants, acid apples, etc., should always be taken an hour after starches (cereals, and all things made from flour, potatoes, rice, etc.).

Quantity, in my view, is as important as quality.

MEAL NO. 2. A SPECIAL VEGETABLE SALAD. This was taken either at breakfast, mid-day or evening. Through this the important chlorophyll was added to the food.

I had some well-washed leaves of spinach, spinach beet, green leaves of lettuce, soft greens of silver beet, as desired, cut up roughly on a wooden chopping board. Then I took a smallish onion, or part of a bigger onion, and cut it up roughly on the board, covered it with the roughly cut-up green leaves (spinach is the best leaf) and applied a very light meat chopper. I chopped it as fine as I would chop mint for mint sauce. After the first month, I added a dozen well-washed sultanas or raisins and chopped them too. I took a carrot, scarped and washed it and grated it with a good grater.

I mixed the grated carrot and other items together in a básin, to which I added a cut-up tomato (second month) or half an apple, and a dessertspoon of Stock Vinegar. Or I made a little dressing of Stock Vinegar, say, a table-spoonful and six dates cut up, with a tablespoon of milk, and a teaspoonful of corn or olive, or sunflower oil. This is roughly the quantity of dressing needed for a breakfast cup of the chopped green salad. I had this special chopped vegetable salad with a cooked vegetable meal or on porridge (a big tablespoonful), or with brown salt-free bread and salt-free butter, or by itself with half a cup of hot water.

This chlorophyll salad is very nice and wholesome, and I took it daily. It is wonderfully purifying, and is a sure, gentle laxative.

MEAL NO. 3. COOKED VEGETABLE MEAL. Breakfast or mid-day or evening. I cooked the vegetables in one of the following ways:

1. Conservatively: that is, with as much of the minerals retained in them as possible.
2. As puree, in which several vegetables are cooked together in one pot, to a thick mush. All the minerals are retained in them.

But, whichever way I chose, I found the addition of raw salad to the meal was necessary. I took a mixture of salad vegetables from grated carrot, parsley, tender celery stalks, raw beet, mint, thyme, mustard and cress, water cress, lettuce, and the green leaves of silver beet and celery.

The raw vegetables provided me with the vitamins, and cooked vegetables with the minerals.

CONSERVATIVE COOKING

For conservative cooking there are several ways. The aim is for the vegetables when cooked to have no, or very little, liquid remaining. I roasted potatoes in their jackets and cooked vegetables in a Pyrex dish, or in parchment paper, or in a double saucepan, or in a covered basin placed inside a saucepan of water to boil. The vegetables were not allowed to overcook to any degree.

Pressure cookers are good for cooking hard vegetables, such as dried beans or peas, but they are not the best for soft vegetables. It is so hard not to overcook with them, and they are not always lined with steel or tin. If they are made of aluminium I found it wise to prevent any chance of metal contamination by putting the vegetables in a covered enamel basin which is then placed inside the cooker. I found another way of conservative cooking was to grease the bottom of an enamel frying pan, and place the vegetables in. I covered them with an enamel plate, and added spoonfuls of water from time to time, until the vegetables were deliciously cooked.

By a little study I was able to make vegetarian cookery very delicious, even without table salt. A good diet reform cookery book,* is of invaluable help.

Another way of conservative cooking I used was to grease the bottom of an enamel pot with fat or oil (peanut and corn oil are especially good). I put in the vegetables and placed the pot over an element turned up to top heat. At once I added a cup of hot water and turned the element down low and then cooked. If need be, I lifted the lid from time to time and added tablespoons of hot water.

* *Everywoman's Wholefood Cook Book* by Vivien Quick, is very good. Obtain from the publishers of this book

Often this was not necessary. When cooked, there was not more than a tablespoon of moisture. Then I dished up and added my chlorophyll salad. This way produced a particularly delicious meal.

One must always have some protein vegetable with these meals, such as cooked peas or dried beans. Where the liver or digestive organs are not affected by cancer one may have an egg, or unsalted cream cheese, with this meal, in the third month, for the protein. Eggs to be eaten not more frequently than every second day.

The puree way I prepared vegetables was a little different. When the vegetables were reduced to a mush in an enamel saucepan, I added half to one tablespoon of soya bean flour, per person, and then thickened with a little pea flour, which had been mixed with cold water and simmered for ten minutes at the least. I dished up and added the chlorophyll salad. As vegetables have no natural oil, like meat, a teaspoon of oil, for each person, was added at the beginning. One should have at least a dessertspoon of oil, such as oilive, soya bean, corn, or sunflower oil, daily.

One very severely ill patient with cancer of the liver, progressed wonderfully by having porridge with chopped raw spinach added for breakfast, vegetables for lunch, as described (alternating the methods), and merely lettuce leaves, spring onions, radishes and salt-free bread and butter for tea, with frequent teaspoons of Stock Vinegar in food and drink during the day. When they can be obtained, salt-free Granose biscuits, also salt-free peanut butter are good.

SUBSTITUTES FOR ANIMAL MEAT are (1) Nuts (I took them daily) and (2) Legumes (I took them daily) such as peas, beans, chestnuts, lentils, pea flour, soya bean flour, linseed (or millet seed, for a change), gluten meal, and unsalted peanut butter. Soya bean flour is the best of all proteins. I made sure that it was fresh when I bought it, and kept it in a glass jar with a lid. I put two to three teaspoons of it in porridge, or bread and milk, or stirred two to three teaspoons in a hot drink.

Pea flour requires a little cooking. Any edible seeds, such as sunflower, are equivalent to a legume. I found Canadian wonder beans were good. I took ample unsalted pure butter with vegetables, and a little acidulated milk or a tablespoon of *pure,* unsalted cream. The third month I took a slice of *very mild* cheese alternately with the egg days.

I kept out of doors or in the *fresh air* and *sunshine* all I could. I always kept *warm,* especially my *feet,* and I practised deep breathing daily. If in winter the chlorophyll salad seemed too cold, I took it warm (*warm only*) by putting it in with the hot vegetables. Another way was to butter and cut up, in squares, a slice of bread and put in an enamel saucepan with a little acidulated milk and water, or acidulated milk and vegetable water (water vegetables cooked in) and bring to the boil. I took it off the heat and droped salad in, and stirred. I put it in a little basin, and chewed it well. I found it best to add some cooked vegetables to this dish before I put in the salad. I found very mild cheese good *after* the tenth week.

I made sure never to cook in aluminium saucepans. Aluminium is not poisonous, but the *lead* with it is amalgamated may be harmful.

NEVER, NEVER FORGET that cancer is due to excessive sodium in 99 per cent of cases, plus a debilitated constitution, through breaking the Laws of Good Health described in Chapter XVIII.

All through this book I have tried to impress upon readers that in cancer the patient's constitution was debilitated *before* he or she developed the disease, because his or her system succumbed to the excess of sodium, and by describing my own cure, I hope I have shown that such an excess can be countered and sufferers restored to good health.

It was about twelve years ago when it was discovered that I myself was suffering from cancer of the bowel, and experiencing the intense pain of the disease. My best plan of action, I felt, was to seek the assistance of a lady patient whom I had cured earlier of cancer. I felt that she would be suited to help me, having been through the mill herself.

She kept me in bed eight weeks, and two months of treatment as outlined in this chapter were undertaken in order to restore the sodium balance of my system.

At this period of the treatment I felt I was a bag of sore bones. Every moment was agonizing, but I knew I must not complain. In spite of the continuing, but gradually lessening, pain, I knew I was getting better.

It is here that I want to emphasize that it required as long as *nearly two years before complete cure was established beyond doubt.*

I have remained entirely free of the disease ever since. *Needless to say, I have adhered religiously to my beliefs as expressed throughout this book.*

Other recommended books...
AN END TO CANCER?
A NUTRITIONAL APPROACH TO ITS PREVENTION AND CONTROL

Leon Chaitow, N.D., D.O. A total biological approach to the treatment of cancer, combining a dietetic regime, vitamin therapy (including vitamin B17, from which Laetrile is derived), enzyme and mineral therapy, and psychotherapy. The facts presented are supported by scrupulous research and there is a glossary of technical terms enabling all laymen to understand fully this revolutionary approach to the problem of cancer. *Contents include:* How cancer starts; Edible, medical and industrial carcinogens; Laetrile and cancer; Prohibited foods; Recommended foods; Outward signs of a pre-cancerous condition; Supplements for the cancer patient; The orthodox treatment of cancer; Psychological considerations—the reality and value of hope.

ABOUT LAETRILE
VITAMIN B17 AND THE FIGHT AGAINST CANCER

Leon Chaitow N.D., D.O. Tells the amazing and inspiring history of this concentrated form of a naturally occurring substance—vitamin B17, now believed to be effective in cancer therapy. Vitamin B17 is found in apricot and peach kernels, bitter almonds, elderberries, wild blackberries and raspberries. The book contains a chapter on the great Laetrile controversy which reveals the harassment suffered by American doctors who prescribed Laetrile for their cancer patients. But Laetrile is non-toxic, is not a drug, and if present in a balanced diet in sufficient quantity, it offers real protection against cancer.

CANCER PREVENTION
FALLACIES AND SOME REASSURING FACTS

Cyril Scott. The mere mention of the word 'cancer' is often sufficient to evoke an atmosphere of fear and terror, but this sane and intelligent book removes a lot of the dread born of the many misunderstandings surrounding the subject. Cyril Scott reviews various theories relating to the origin of the disease, enumerates recoveries attributed to naturopathic, homoeopathic and biochemic treatments, and presents his own conclusions. He also offers details of a simple preventive measure which will reassure every reader. *Contents include:* Homoepathic achievements; The meat-eating habit; Effects of prolonged worry; The grape cure; Potassium foods; Iron foods; Honey—a perfect food and polychrest.

THE COMPLETE RAW JUICE THERAPY

Susan E. Charmine. Most comprehensive guide ever published on the healing and regenerative powers of energy-packed raw juices—which contain high concentrations of vitamins, minerals, *natural* sugars and enzymes. When the cells of freshly picked plants are 'unlocked' this goodness is released as pure liquids of great healing value. The gentle action of juices can strengthen the functioning of our bodies and coax them back to normality when they are below par, without risk of side-effects. Author provides an alphabetical list of ailments with exact dosages of appropriate juice remedies and explains exactly how raw juice therapy works.

VITAMINS
WHAT THEY ARE AND WHY WE NEED THEM

Carol Hunter. Explains the characteristics of all known vitamins, their role in health and nutrition, the deficiency symptoms that occur when they are not found in the diet. Includes chapters on improving one's appearance, individual vitamin needs, minimizing vitamin loss in cooking, and megavitamin therapy for alcoholism, schizophrenia, and other diseases. *Other contents:* The discovery of Niacin; E for fertility; Where to find vitamin A; Spotting a deficiency; The role of Thiamine; Why we need vitamin C; Assessing your requirements; Brewer's yeast for B vitamins; The value of wheat germ; Molasses—a nutritious sweetener; Growing your own bean sprouts; Planning your own daily diet.

ABOUT DEVIL'S CLAW
ARTHRITIS REMEDY FROM AFRICA

Maurice Hanssen. Reveals the amazing story of Devil's Claw, a plant which grows wild on the South West African steppes and in the Kalahari Desert. The seeds of the plant are secreted in a claw-like pod which is extremely tough, with a propensity for gripping anything making contact with it. For centuries in Africa Devil's Claw has been known for its revitalizing effect on muscles and joints, and it is now marketed as tablets and teas for treating arthritis, rheumatism and gout. Devil's Claw also alleviates poor circulation of the blood, back sores, indigestion and nervous stomach disorders, gall bladder, intestinal and kidney complaints.

THE RAW FOOD WAY TO HEALTH
CHANGE YOUR EATING HABITS AND CHANGE YOUR LIFE

Janet Hunt. Raw is healthy! Good health, says the author, is something we all want; and yet our modern life-style with its scientifically produced convenience foods does little to encourage healthy living. But by adopting a raw food diet the body is supplied with all the vitamins, minerals and roughage it needs in a way it can easily assimilate. The author gives a list of delicious salad combinations to show that raw food living need not be a dreary, unimaginative process. Also includes: raw food as a cure for common ailments, home-growing, buying raw food.

ALTERNATIVE COOKING
A TREASURY OF NUTRITIOUS AND UNUSUAL RECIPES

Greet Buchner. Fascinating collection of nutritious recipes using wild and cultivated vegetables—and what are commonly regarded as weeds. Explains how to make Stinging nettle soup, Stewed coltsfoot, Chickweed salad, Dandelion salad, Rose honey, Elder blossom fritters, Shepherd's purse soup, and other delicacies. There are also original recipes using potatoes, mushrooms, rice and nuts. Alternative cooking means following the natural cycle of the seasons, gathering berries in autumn, for example, or making use of the tender leaves of dandelions in spring. There is also a chapter on biodynamics—the theory that plants effect a direct influence on man's spiritual as well as physical well-being.

FREE FOR ALL

Weeds as a Source of Food

Ceres. *Illustrated.* All around us—in fields, woods and hedgerows—there are wild plants free for the picking, many highly nutritious, some with specific medicinal uses. An experienced naturalist and botanical writer here describes about 150 of these plants, where and when to find them, prepare, cook and store them. Includes information on acorns, alfalfa, beefsteak fungus, butcher's broom, cauliflower toadstool, charlock, hedge garlic, nettle, puffball, and other edible 'weeds'—with a section on poisonous plants to be avoided.

ABOUT GINSENG

The Magical Herb of the East

Stephen Fulder, M.A., Ph.D. Ginseng, the strange 'man-shaped' root of the Orient, has been used as a panacea for thousands of years in the East. Now it is freely available in the West, notably from health food stores, and Stephen Fulder explains exactly where and how Ginseng is cultivated; the different forms available; its effect on the ageing process; its value in treating cardiovascular disease, sexual impotence, depression, insomnia, and many other conditions. *Part contents:* Ginseng and herbal medicine in China; Ginseng as stimulant and sedative; Ginseng and potency; What does Ginseng contain?; How to take Ginseng; Ginseng today.

HERBAL TEAS FOR HEALTH AND HEALING

Ceres. *Illustrated.* Over a hundred tea-making herbs are described in this delightful book. Some are slightly stimulating, others are tonics for restoring the system to complete health. Many can 'lift' melancholy and depression; others are nocturnal and daytime tranquillizers, and there are teas to alleviate pain and clear the skin, also herbal infusions for external uses as poultices and skin-tonics. *Includes:* Carminative teas 'for comforting the stomacke'; Cosmetic teas 'for helping to beautify the skin'; Pain-killing teas 'for allaying the agony'; Febrifuge teas 'to allay the fever'; Teas to induce sleep 'and to help settle obstreporous spirits'.

PROVEN REMEDIES

The Treatment of Common Ailments by Homoeopathic, Herbal & Biochemic Methods

J. H. Oliver N.A.M.H. All these remedies are more genuinely scientific than drugs. The latter come and go, being first acclaimed and often ultimately discredited. But the herb and plant remedies endure: 'what cured a hundred years ago still cures today.' Here is a large number of alphabetically listed ailments, with the corresponding remedies and precise instructions as to dosage. In some cases osteopathy or chiropractic is also recommended and J. H. Oliver has added some valuable notes on deficiency foods, natural food, vitamins and germs.

BEYOND THE STAFF OF LIFE
A WHEATLESS, DAIRYLESS, VEGETARIAN COOKBOOK

Kief Adler. For the venturesome, this book is a splendid means through which to experience the delights of exotic cuisines. It is a godsend for persons allergic to wheat, milk, salt, etc. Sufferers from multiple sclerosis find here a diet that nourishes superbly, while excluding their principal bane—the gluten of wheat. The cookbook, which will add a new dimension to your culinary capabilities, was researched and written by a young chef who has personally explored the cuisines of North Africa, the Middle and Far East. It is based on really up-to-date nutritional knowledge and contains a wealth of healthful recipes for everyone.

SECRETS OF THE CHINESE HERBALISTS

Richard Lucas. Safe, effective Chinese herbal formulas for treating circulatory disorders, bowel complaints, respiratory ailments, urinary problems, insomnia, sex complications, prostate trouble, hay fever, female irregularities, and many other ills. There is also an entire chapter on fabulous Ginseng, the sex rejuvenant and longevity plant, prized for thousands of years in the Orient as a specific for numerous ailments. Author's task included sifting through volumes of Oriental herb writings and undertaking lengthy in-depth consultations with many Chinese practitioners. In fact, he researched the background, history and medical use of Chinese herbs for over twenty years before writing this book.

ABOUT BIOCHEMIC SALTS
WITH AN EXPLANATION OF THE TWELVE TISSUE SALTS, A NUTRITIONAL THERAPY INVOLVING MICRO-NUTRIENTS

Esther Chapman. 'Biochemistry' means the chemistry of living tissues. This book explains the elements that have formed the earth and human bodies, and which are essential for health and intelligence. *Contents include:* The earth's elements become human tissue cells; The metabolism of cells—endocrine glands—the respiratory and alimentary systems; Digestion and absorption of food—chemical activities within human tissues—the oxidation process—osmosis; Adult nutritional balances—daily food requirements based on calories—the vitamins; The Twelve Tissue Salts used in nutritional therapy—some uses for each of the salts.

ACUPUNCTURE ENERGY IN HEALTH AND DISEASE
A PRACTICAL GUIDE FOR ADVANCED STUDENTS

Henry Woollerton, Dr.Ac., & Colleen J. McLean, B.A. *Illustrated.* Containing much information that has not so far been easily available, this book deals with the principles of energy distribution in health and disease, illustrated by detailed line drawings in accordance with Chinese methods of practising the diagnosis of disease. The practical treatments described take five basic forms: Needle acupuncture; Electronic stimulation acupuncture; Needle-less acupuncture; Press needle and dermal needle therapy. There are also chapters on moxibustion and on the rapidly developing practice of electronic acupuncture.

THE ACUPUNCTURE TREATMENT OF PAIN

Leon Chaitow. *Large format. Over 200 diagrams.* For all who practise pain relief—doctors, surgeons, osteopaths, chiropractors, physiotherapists, trained nurses—this book shows how to apply the analgesic (pain relieving) and anaesthetic benefits of acupuncture with maximum efficacy, The location and anatomical position of each point is clearly described and given its Chinese name, traditional meridian name, and number. This information is adjacent to detailed, two-colour diagrams, thus enabling each point to be found with ease and accuracy. Author studied acupuncture under Dr J. Lavier, and since 1966 he has researched into the usefulness of acupuncture for pain relief.

BRAN

HOW BRAN REPLACES FIBRE MISSING FROM TODAY'S DIET, THUS ELIMINATING CONSTIPATION AND COLONIC DISEASES

Ray Hill. Apart from relieving constipation and other bowel disorders, such as colitis and diverticulitis, bran also fulfils an important function in the slimming diet which is both physical and psychological in that it creates in a meal bulk which is not absorbed by the body. This book shows how to use bran in the daily preparation of meals, and there are a number of tasty recipes for bran breads, biscuits, scones and puddings; plus a selection of bran breakfast ideas, bran drinks, and even bran for the skin.

ABOUT FASTING

A ROYAL ROAD TO HEALING AND IDEAL METHOD OF TREATMENT FOR THE WHOLE BODY SYSTEM

Otto H. F. Buchinger M.D. Explains in simple terms the benefits to be derived from a healing fast for the recovery and regeneration of body, mind and spirit. That fasting is a natural reaction to illness is proved by the fact that one of the first symptoms of the onset of an acute disease is loss of appetite! *Contents include:* Overweight and rheumatism; Heart and circulatory disorders; How the fasting treatment is carried out; Bodily care during the fasting days; Rest, exercise and health education; Digestive and other disorders; Diet plan.

ARTHRITIS Help in Your Own Hands

Helen B. MacFarlane. No one, however 'crippled' by chronic arthritis, need wait impotently for the disease to complete its destructive work. Author progressed from semi-invalidism to mobility through practising techniques—explained in this book—which are designed to stop deterioration and activate the healing process! Her success could be applied to almost anyone suffering from osteoarthritis, fibrositis, or other rheumatic diseases. *Contents include:* Electric massagers; Exercises; Vitamin deficiencies; Cortisone-producing diet; Importance of moderation; Connection between arthritis and 'negative personality'; The 'rheumatoid factor'; Ionizers; Cultured milk; minerals; Cod liver oil therapy; Fats; Helpful organizations; Aids and appliances; Useful hints.

EVERYBODY'S GUIDE TO NATURE CURE

The most comprehensive treatise on Nature Cure that has ever been published containing 486 pages of unrivalled health knowledge. Part 1 deals with Nature Cure in Theory and Outline. Part 2 describes fully the self-treatment of Child Ailments, Diseases of the Skin and Scalp; Joints and Rheumatic Affections; The Blood, Blood-Vessels and Circulatory System; Nerves and Nervous System; Eyes; Ears, Nose. Mouth and Throat; Stomach and Intestines; Heart Lungs, Bronchial Tubes, and Larynx; Liver, Gall-Bladder, Kidneys, Bladder and Pancreas; Male and Female Sex Organs. Deals with Fevers and Influenza and contains General Treatments, Diets, First-Aid etc.—and is comprehensively indexed for easy reference.

KELP FOR BETTER HEALTH AND VITALITY

NOURISHING FOOD FROM SEAWEED

Frank Wilson. Explains the nutritional and medicinal benefits of kelp and other seaweeds. There are some 800 varieties around the shores of the British Isles alone, most of them representing a substantial nutritional resource. Kelp in particular contains a wide range of essential vitamins, minerals and trace elements. In Wales, Ireland and Scotland seaweed was a traditional food; in Europe it was utilized as fertilizer, potash and iodine. Unusual recipes include: Sprout and Seaweed soup; Kombu fry; Dulse and Fruit salad.

ACUPRESSURE TECHNIQUES

FOR THE SELF-TREATMENT OF MINOR AILMENTS

Dr Hans Ewald. *Illustrated.* Acupressure was developed from the Chinese healing system of acupuncture. It makes use of the same points and meridians (paths), but thumbs and forefingers are used instead of needles. Its prime use is in alleviating and healing nervous diseases, with particular reference to nervous exhaustion, anxiety states, heart and circulatory disturbances, impotence, frigidity, insomnia, headaches, and skin complaints. The technique is explained lucidly in this excellent handbook. Pictures and supplementary drawings indicate the exact location of the points, which should be activated in a clockwise direction for between one and five minutes. Beneficial reaction is quick and lasts for some time.

CHINESE MICRO-MASSAGE

Acupuncture Without Needles

J. Lavier. *Illustrated.* The areas massaged in Chinese micro-massage are cutaneous zones of less than a square centimetre. They are activated by the thumb tips instead of needles. Author fully explains a fascinating therapy that bridges the gap between classical massage and acupuncture. Micro-massage is an *energizing* action, resembling the application of small electrodes to the 'motor points' of muscles. It is used on children and squeamish adults who are afraid of the acupuncture needles. Previously published descriptions of micro-massage have been—at best—fragments of source works; this book is a complete explanation of the therapy.